MODERN CHINESE ACUPUNCTURE

An up-to-date view of acupuncture techniques as being practised in China today, including new developments and advice on the treatment of some common diseases.

DEDICATION
To our Chinese friends and teachers.

MODERN CHINESE ACUPUNCTURE

by
G. T. LEWITH, M.A., M.R.C.G.P., M.R.C.P.
and
N. R. LEWITH, M.C.S.P.

THORSONS PUBLISHERS LIMITED
Wellingborough, Northamptonshire
THORSONS PUBLISHERS INC.
New York

First published 1980
Second edition, revised and reset, 1983

British Library Cataloguing in Publication Data

Lewith, G. T.
  Modern Chinese acupuncture
  1. Acupuncture — China — History
  — 20th century
  I. Title   II. Lewith, N. R.
  615'.892'0951   RM184
  ISBN 0-7225-0924-3

*Thorsons Publishers Inc. are distributed to the trade by
Inner Traditions International Ltd.,
377 Park Avenue South, New York, NY 10016.*

Printed and bound in Great Britain

CONTENTS

ACKNOWLEDGEMENT
We should like to thank Constance Knight
for her excellent work on the manuscript.

PREFACE TO
THE SECOND EDITION

This second edition of *Modern Chinese Acupuncture* provides further useful information about traditional Chinese medicine and also updates some of the current physiological explanations for acupuncture. The basic principles of traditional Chinese medicine have been expanded to include 'The Differentiation of Syndromes'. The reader is advised to use this new material as a reference rather than attempting to memorize all the minutiae of each syndrome. It is important to remember that the basic concepts of traditional Chinese medicine are of over-riding importance, and details are only of value if the reader already understands these principles. The addition of this section completes the picture of the traditional Chinese approach to acupuncture as it is currently taught in China, and will also allow the reader to obtain a more profound grasp of specific organ function.

The last section of the book on the physiological mechanisms of acupuncture has been updated as a considerable amount of new work has been published in this field over the last three or four years. The authors hope that this text will continue to provide acupuncturists with a useful and practical reference to the modern teaching of traditional Chinese medicine.

G. T. AND N. R. LEWITH, 1983.

INTRODUCTION

This book is based on the lectures we attended while on an acupuncture course at the College of Traditional Chinese Medicine at Nanking in China, and it represents the way the Chinese are thinking about acupuncture at the moment. We do not discuss the actual location of acupuncture points as this information is available from such books as *An Outline of Chinese Acupuncture* published by the Foreign Languages Press in Peking. In our book we have used the Chinese names and numbering system.

It is very simple to learn and use a basic form of acupuncture for the treatment of pain, but it is vital to understand the principles of traditional medicine in order to be most effective, and to treat internal diseases such as asthma. The present work on pain goes some way towards explaining the mechanism of acupuncture, but at the moment the scientific approach to acupuncture does not tell us which point to select for a particular problem. We do not decry the scientific approach to acupuncture, quite the contrary; ultimately it may indicate a more physiological approach to point selection, but at the moment such indication is not available. It seems logical, then, that until it is available we should use the empirical clinical experience that has been obtained from many centuries of work by the Chinese.

The Chinese have rationalized their clinical experience into a detailed system and, by using this system, the acupuncturist can benefit from their experience and obtain better therapeutic results. In China there is no conflict between the traditional and scientific approaches: it is realized that both are being used for the benefit of the patient and that both are developing different aspects of the same problem. We feel that this attitude of mutual acceptance is vital if this therapy is to progress.

We have divided the book into five main sections. The Basic Principles of Traditional Chinese Medicine deals with the traditional Chinese approach to health and disease; the second section on The Principles of Therapy describes how this approach should be used to select acupuncture points for a particular disease. The third section discusses some common diseases and their treatment. The fourth and fifth sections are more modern additions to acupuncture therapy; the fourth section dealing with ear, scalp and hand acupuncture, and the fifth dealing with acupuncture anaesthesia and the scientific basis of acupuncture.

The sections on traditional Chinese medicine are a modern Chinese version of traditional medicine. They have simplified and adapted the many complex rules of classical Chinese medicine so that they are usable and understandable. Even so it may be quite difficult for a Westerner to understand these ideas at first glance, and we suggest that the reader quickly reads through Sections 1 and 2 to get an idea of the contents, and then re-reads these sections more thoroughly.

In spite of this simplified approach to traditional Chinese medicine all the major traditional philosophical concepts are integrated into this system. We feel that this modern adaptation of classical Chinese medicine has lost nothing in terms of therapeutic benefit to the patient, and has gained a great deal in making the concepts more universally understandable.

Acupuncture is a clinical discipline and no book can replace clinical experience. However, we feel that this book is an important resource for acupuncturists and members of the lay public who are interested in acupuncture.

THE BASIC PRINCIPLES OF CHINESE TRADITIONAL MEDICINE

I. YIN AND YANG

The theory of yin and yang is a kind of world outlook. It holds that all things have two opposite aspects, yin and yang, which are both opposite and at the same time interdependent. This is a universal law of the material world. These two aspects are in opposition to each other but because one end of the spectrum cannot exist without the other they are interdependent.

The ancient Chinese used water and fire to symbolize yin and yang; anything moving, hot, bright and hyperactive is yang, and anything quiescent, cold, dim and hypoactive is yin.

The yin and yang properties of things are not absolute but relative. As an object or person changes so the yin and yang components change at a gradual rate. Each of the yin and yang properties of the object is a condition for the existence of the other; neither can exist in isolation.

These two opposites are not stationary but in constant motion. If we imagine the circadian rhythm, night is yin and day is yang; as night (yin) fades it becomes day (yang), and as yang fades it becomes yin. Yin and yang are therefore changing into each other as well as balancing each other.

The Application of Yin and Yang to Chinese Medicine
Each organ has an element of yin and yang within it. The histological structures and nutrients are yin, and the functional

DAY YANG

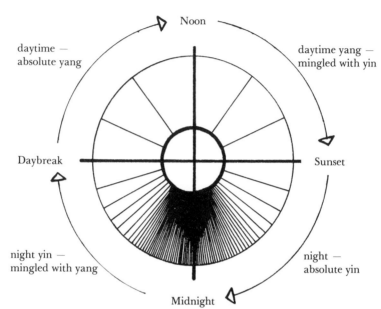

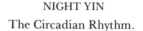

NIGHT YIN

The Circadian Rhythm.

activities are yang. Some organs are predominantly yang in their functions, such as the gan-liver, while others are predominantly yin, such as the shen-kidney. Even though one organ may be predominantly yin (or yang) in nature, the balance of yin and yang is maintained in the whole healthy body because the sum total of the yin and yang will be in a fluctuating balance.

If a condition of prolonged excess or deficiency of either yin or yang occurs then disease results. In an excess of yin the yang qi[1] would be damaged, and a disease of cold of shi[1] nature would develop. Excess of yang will consume yin and a disease of heat of shi nature would develop. In a deficiency of yin, diseases of heat of xu[1] nature develop, while a deficiency of yang causes diseases of cold of xu nature.

[1] The concept of qi is explained on page 20, shi on page 27 and xu on page 27.

Hyperactivity of yin —
injures yang

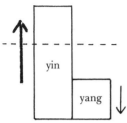

disease of cold of shi nature
(yin in excess produces cold)

Hyperactivity of yang —
injures yin

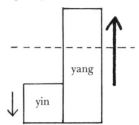

disease of heat of shi nature
(yang in excess produces heat)

Hypoactivity of yin —
leads to hyperactivity of yang

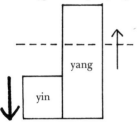

disease of heat of xu nature

Hypoactivity of yang —
leads to hyperactivity of yin

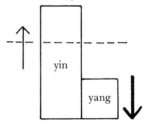

disease of cold of xu nature

Hyperactivity and Hypoactivity of Yin and Yang.

II. THE CHANNELS AND COLLATERALS

The channels and collaterals are the representation of the organs of the body. They are also a functional system in their own right and they are responsible for conducting the flow of qi and blood through the body. The flow of qi can be disrupted by direct damage to the channels, such as trauma, or by an internal imbalance of yin and yang within the body.

The central principle of traditional Chinese medicine is to diagnose the cause of the internal disease, or yin yang imbalance within the body, and, by using the relevant acupuncture points, to correct the flow of qi in the channels and thus correct the internal disease. The acupuncture points that are on the channels have a direct influence on the flow of qi through the channels, and also on the internal organs. The zang channels are yin in nature and the fu channels are yang in nature.

Qi circulates through the channels of the body in a well defined circadian rhythm.

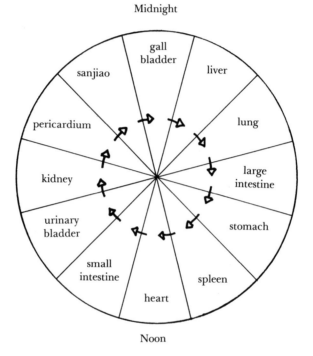

The Circulation of Qi.

III. ZANG AND FU ORGANS

The zang and fu organs are the internal visible organs of the body. The xin-heart, gan-liver, pi-spleen, fei-lung, shen-kidney and pericardium are the zang organs. The small intestine, large intestine, stomach, gall-bladder, urinary bladder and sanjiao are the fu organs.

The zang organs have a Chinese prefix because a direct translation from the Chinese might be misleading. The Chinese xin has functions rather different from the concept of the heart in

Western medicine, so if we call the heart 'xin-heart', or the liver 'gan-liver', we are able to understand that we are referring to the organ of the heart or the liver, but it is really rather different from our concept of those organs.

The zang organs are of paramount importance in the body. They co-ordinate with the fu organs and connect with the five tissues (channels, jin,[2] muscles, skin-hair, bones), and the nine openings (eyes, nose, ears, mouth, tongue, anus and external genitalia), to form the system of the Five Zang. The pericardium is not considered to be an important zang organ.

The Functions of the Zang Organs

The xin-heart

The xin-heart dominates the circulation of blood. When it functions properly the tissues and organs are well perfused and nourished, but when it malfunctions there is precordial pain, cyanosis and ischaemia. This disease is due to 'stagnation of the blood of xin-heart'.

The xin-heart 'keeps' the mind. Normally there is a clear mind, normal mentality, normal sleep and a good memory. When this fails there is coma, insomnia or somnolence, amnesia and mental derangement, because the xin-heart is failing to 'keep' the mind.

The xin-heart takes the tongue as its orifice and opens through it. Normally the tongue is reddish, moist, and moves freely. When the tongue has ulcers, is swollen or becomes purplish-red, there is 'upward blazing of the fire in xin-heart'. When the tongue is rigid and curled up (this may be accompanied by mental symptoms) 'phlegm and heat are covering the orifice of the xin-heart'.

The gan-liver

The gan-liver is the main yang organ of the body.

The gan-liver stores blood. Normally there is sufficient blood supply to all tissues. When this fails there is ischaemia, dizziness, malaise, abnormal menstruation and haemorrhage.

The gan-liver takes charge of freeing. Freeing really means the free flow of blood and qi through the body, especially digestion and the discharge of bile. When this is impaired there is irrit-

[2]Jin is a tissue that is composed of nerves, ligaments, tendons and some parts of the muscle. It is roughly equivalent to connective tissue.

ability, mental depression, anorexia, abdominal distension and jaundice.

The gan-liver controls the jin which governs the muscle tone. When this function is disturbed there is muscle spasm, twitching, opisthotonos and convulsions. This is due to an 'insufficiency of yin and blood of the gan-liver, resulting in the malnutrition of the jin'.

The gan-liver takes the eye as its orifice and opens through it. Usually there is normal vision and normal eye movement. When this function is disturbed there is poor vision, night blindness, nystagmus and abnormal eye movements. This is due to an 'insufficiency of yin and blood in the gan-liver causing malnutrition of the eyes and stirring of the inner wind of the gan-liver.'

The pi-spleen

The pi-spleen governs the transportation and transformation of food, i.e. digestion. When digestion is abnormal there is anorexia, distension of the abdomen, diarrhoea, emaciation, lassitude and oedema. This is due to 'a deficiency of the qi of pi-spleen'.

The pi-spleen commands the blood. Normally the blood circulates within the blood vessels but when this function fails there is extravasation of blood, chronic recurrent haemorrhage and bruising.

The pi-spleen dominates the muscles. This really means controlling the muscle bulk. Normally there is no muscle wasting, but when there is malnutrition of the muscles they are weak and wasted.

The pi-spleen takes the mouth as its orifice and opens through it. Normal people have a good appetite, a sense of smell and taste and red and moist lips. Abnormally there is anorexia, tastelessness or a sweetish, greasy taste, and pale sore lips. This is due to 'heat and damp in the pi-spleen'.

In addition the qi of pi-spleen lifts and fixes the internal organs in their normal position.

The fei-lung

The fei-lung takes charge of respiration. Normally respiration is even and the tissues are well oxygenated. When this function fails breathing is uneven, there is a cough, dyspnoea, shallow respiration and anoxia. This is due to 'a deficiency of qi of fei-lung which causes an impairment of dissipation and descent of clean qi (oxygen)'.

The fei-lung frees and regulates the water passage. This function covers the transportation and distribution of nutrients and water, the secretion of sweat and the excretion of urine. Abnormally there will be hyperhydrosis or hypohydrosis, oedema and difficulty in urination due to 'obstruction of the water passage'.

The fei-lung dominates the hair and skin. Normally the skin is lubricious, the hair lustrous, and sweating is normal. Abnormally the skin is rough, the hair dry and withered and the skin is 'loose'. This looseness opens the pores and increases the susceptibility to invasion by pathogenic factors.

The fei-lung takes the nose as its orifice and opens through it. Normally the nose is open and there is an acute sense of smell. Abnormally it may be obstructed, there may be anosmia, epistaxis and flaring of the alae nasi (usually accompanied by fever). This is due to 'invasion of the fei-lung by wind and cold or wind and heat'.

The shen-kidney

The shen-kidney is the main yin organ of the body. The shen-kidney dominates growth, reproduction and development. When this function fails there is a loss of reproductive function, retardation of growth, failure to thrive, and premature senility due to 'an insufficiency of the qi of shen-kidney'.

The shen-kidney produces marrow, filling the brain with marrow, dominating the bones and producing blood. Normally the spinal cord and the brain are fully developed, the bones are strong and the blood sufficient. Abnormally there will be dizziness, tinnitus, insomnia, poor memory and lassitude. The bones will be weak and brittle and the blood will be insufficient. This is due to 'an insufficiency of the essence of shen-kidney'.

The shen-kidney controls body water. This entails normal urine production and micturition. Abnormally there will be oliguria or anuria, oedema, difficult or dribbling micturition, polyuria, enuresis and incontinence. This is due to 'an insufficiency of yang of the shen-kidney failing to control body water'.

The shen-kidney controls the intake of clean qi (air). Abnormally there will be wheezing due to 'the failure of the shen-kidney to control the intake of clean air'.

The shen-kidney takes the ear as its orifice, opening through it. Normally there is sharp hearing, abnormally there is tinnitus, hearing loss, and even total deafness.

The pericardium

This may be called the organ of circulation in some texts. It is the least important of the zang organs.

It encloses and protects the xin-heart and the diseases of the pericardium result in dysfunction of the xin-heart.

The Functions of the Fu Organs

In general the traditional functions of the fu organs are very similar to their functions in Western medicine. Each fu organ channel connects internally and externally with a zang organ channel. This can have therapeutic importance in that a point on the fu channel may be used to treat a problem on its connected zang channel, and vice versa.

The small intestine

The small intestine connects with the xin-heart. The small intestine receives and digests food from the stomach. It absorbs the pure part and distributes it to the whole body, the impure part going on to the large intestine. This function of the small intestine belongs to the transforming and transporting function of the pi-spleen.

The gall-bladder

The gall-bladder connects with the gan-liver. It stores and discharges bile. The expulsion of bile from the gall-bladder is closely related to the freeing function of the gan-liver. The gan-liver and the gall-bladder take charge of freeing together, and jaundice results when this function is deranged.

The stomach

The stomach connects with the pi-spleen. The stomach stores and digests food, passing it on to the small intestine. A deficiency of qi of the stomach causes indigestion, epigastric pain and sour regurgitation. When the qi of the stomach ascends then nausea, heartburn, vomiting, hiccoughs and flatulence occur.

The large intestine

The large intestine connects with the fei-lung. The large intestine absorbs the residue of water and turns the rest of the food into faeces. Disturbance of this function results in diarrhoea or constipation due to the 'descent of qi'.

The urinary bladder

The urinary bladder connects with the shen-kidney. The bladder stores and then discharges urine from the body.

The sanjiao

In Chinese the sanjiao means the three cavities. The xin-heart and the fei-lung are in the upper jiao (the chest), and they transport qi and blood to all parts of the body in order to nourish the body. The pi-spleen and stomach are in the middle jiao (the epi-gastrium) and they digest and absorb food. The shen-kidney and bladder are in the lower jiao (the hypogastrium) and they control water metabolism and the storage and excretion of water. The sanjiao is also sometimes called the triple warmer organ. This is because the three body cavities are intended to control the body temperature.

Extra Organs

The brain

The brain is a sea of marrow, i.e. it is an enlarged part of the spinal cord. The shen-kidney produces the marrow that fills the brain. If the essence of shen-kidney is absent then there is inadequate marrow for the brain. In traditional Chinese medicine the function of the mind is included in that of the xin-heart.

The uterus

The function of the uterus is' to control the menstrual cycle, develop the embryo and nourish the foetus. The qi and blood of the channels pass into the uterus through the chong and the ren channels, so that the qi of the body is able to influence the flow and regularity of the menstrual cycle.

IV. QI, BLOOD AND BODY FLUID

Qi, blood and body fluid are important substances and structures in the body. They sustain the vital activities and they nourish the body, thereby keeping the functions of the tissues, organs and channels in good order. The production and circulation of qi and blood also depends on the health of the tissues and organs that are nourished by these substances.

Qi

Qi is a complex concept; it relates to both substance and function. Clean qi (oxygen), waste qi (carbon dioxide) and qi (nutrients) are generally known as material qi, and the existence of material qi is shown by the functional activity of various organs. The function of an organ depends on the functional qi of that organ; for instance, qi of xin-heart or qi of pi-spleen is the vital energy and functional activity of the xin-heart or pi-spleen. The function of an organ, or its functional qi, cannot exist without material qi, and vice versa.

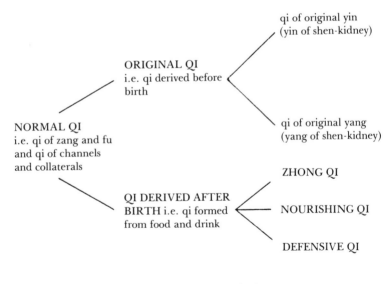

The Constituents of Qi.

Zhong qi

Zhong qi is found mainly in the chest. It nourishes the structures and functions of the xin-heart and fei-lung.

Nourishing qi

Nourishing qi circulates in the channels and collaterals, mainly in the viscera.

Defensive qi

Defensive qi is in the muscles and skin. It circulates outside the channels, in the subcutaneous tissues, and it defends the body against invasion by pathogens.

The original qi is nourished and maintained by qi derived after birth. These combine to form genuine qi, i.e. the total sum of qi in the healthy body. This contrasts with pathogenic factors that are known as pathogenic qi.

Blood

The nutrients from food are digested by the pi-spleen and stomach and they are then transported to the xin-heart and fei-lung and turned into red (oxygenated) blood by qi. The essence of shen-kidney produces bone marrow, and bone marrow uses the digested food to produce blood.

Qi of shen-kidney promotes digestion by pi-spleen, which in turn strengthens the xin-heart and fei-lung. This interaction therefore promotes haemopoesis.

There is a close relationship between qi and blood. The formation and circulation of blood depends on qi, whereas the formation and distribution of qi, as well as the health of the various organs of the body, is dependent on adequate nourishment from the blood. If the flow of blood 'stagnates' the circulation of qi is 'retarded' and, conversely, if the circulation of qi is 'retarded' then the blood flow 'stagnates'.

Body Fluid

Body fluid is formed from food and drink. It exists in the blood, the tissues, and all the body openings and cavities.

V. THE PATHOGENESIS OF DISEASE

In traditional Chinese medicine various elements and other factors cause disease. These are known as pathogenic factors or pathogens. Normally the human body is able to resist pathogens and maintain a healthy balance between the body and the environment. This ability is a function of normal qi, especially the defensive qi.

Disease develops because normal qi is unable to resist the onslaught of the pathogenic qi; if pathogenic qi overwhelms normal qi then a functional disturbance of the body results. The major principle of treating a disease in Chinese medicine is to strengthen and protect normal qi and maintain a healthy body. In ancient China a physician was only paid while his patient was healthy, not while his patient was ill!

Pathogenic Factors

These are divided into three main groups, exogenous pathogens, mental pathogens and various miscellaneous pathogens. 'Phlegm and humour' and 'stagnant blood' are pathological products; once they are formed new pathological changes will ensue so they are considered to be secondary pathogens.

Pathological factors serve as a generalization of clinical symptoms and signs, reflecting the struggle of normal qi and pathogenic qi. By differentiating the clinical symptoms and signs the cause of the disease can be traced, and then treatment can be determined. In order to do this the diseased organs must be defined and the pathogen causing that disease must also be diagnosed. This is called the 'determination of treatment on the basis of the differentiation of a syndrome', and it is the basis of diagnosis and treatment in Chinese medicine.

The Exogenous Pathogens

These refer to six relatively abnormal meteorological conditions; wind, cold, summer heat, damp, dryness and heat (fire, warmth). The diseases caused by these pathogens include most viral, bacterial and protozoal diseases and some 'allergic' conditions such as urticaria.

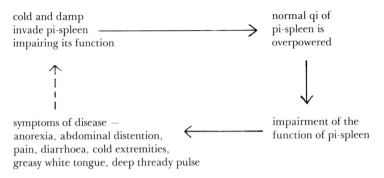

The treatment is to eliminate the cold and damp and strengthen the pi-spleen

The Differentiation of a Syndrome.

Wind

This pathogen is characterized by movability (of symptoms) and changeability. The clinical manifestations are abnormal limb motion, such as spasm or twitching, and a wandering symptomatic site as in urticaria or arthralgia. The symptoms may vary in intensity and they usually include a dislike of wind, fever, sweating, headache and an itchy throat.

Cold

Invasion of cold will consume the yang causing a contraction of the channels and the blood vessels, and therefore a poor circulation of qi and blood. The symptoms are those of a slight fever, a dislike of cold, hypohydrosis, headache, muscular pain and spasm, and occasionally a dark blue and painful area in the local muscles and skin; a frozen shoulder is a good example of the pathogen cold.

Summer heat

This only occurs in the summer; it damages the yin and may progress to affect the level of consciousness. The symptoms are excessive body heat, profuse sweating, thirst, a dry mouth, dry red skin and, in severe cases, delirium (this is known as heat exhaustion in Chinese medicine). Summer heat may combine with wind and cause convulsions. Summer heat often combines with damp to produce dizziness, nausea, a stuffy sensation in the chest and general malaise.

Damp
Diseases caused by damp are sticky, muddy, greasy and stagnant. Damp causes a generalized heavy feeling associated with distension, dizziness and a heavy head, general malaise and a stuffy sensation in the chest. The patient may also complain of abdominal swelling and an exudative and prolonged skin disease.

Dryness
Dryness consumes yin fluid. There may be a dry sore feeling in the nose, mouth and throat, a coarseness of the skin, or a cough with scanty sputum and possibly haemoptysis. Tuberculosis is an example of the pathogen dryness.

Heat (fire, warmth)
All these represent the same pathogen, but at different intensities. Fire is the most severe and warmth the mildest. As with summer heat the yin may be damaged and this will affect the level of consciousness. The main difference is that summer heat only occurs in the summer and is generally less severe than fire. Diseases that are caused by heat are generally of abrupt onset and rapid change, they are nearly always acute infections. Initially the patient may complain of a high fever, chill, thirst, restlessness, irritability and profuse sweating. In severe cases the patient may be in coma with convulsions.

Mental Pathogens

These are overjoy, anger, anxiety, overthinking, grief, fear and fright.

Excessive fear and fright, or overjoy, injures the xin-heart. This causes palpitations, insomnia, irritability, anxiety and mental abnormality.

Excessive anger causes dysfunction of the gan-liver. This impairs the function of freeing, and causes pain and distention in the costal and hypochondriac region, abnormal menstruation, depression and irritability. If the function of storing blood is disturbed then menorrhagia and haemorrhage can result.

Excessive grief, anxiety and overthinking cause dysfunction of the pi-spleen and stomach. This causes anorexia and a feeling of fullness or distension after meals.

Excessive grief, anxiety and anger cause poor circulation of qi and blood. If there is retardation of qi and stagnation of blood then this can cause a tumour.

Miscellaneous Pathogens

Irregular feeding

Overeating, or eating too much uncooked or cold food, impairs the function of pi-spleen and stomach and causes nausea, vomiting, heartburn, sour regurgitation and diarrhoea; for example dyspepsia, gastritis and enteritis.

Over-indulgence in alcohol and an excess of fatty or hot, pungent food produces damp and heat, or phlegm and heat, in the pi-spleen and stomach. Initially dyspepsia results but in more severe cases hypertension, enteritis, gastritis, cirrhosis, cancer or ischaemic heart disease can result. All these are related to nutritional habits.

Too little food intake, or lack of some essential material in food, may cause malnutrition. This results in a deficiency of qi and blood which causes emaciation, lassitude, palpitations and sometimes coma.

The intake of contaminated food may impair the function of pi-spleen and stomach, and cause intestinal infections and various parasitic diseases.

Too little or excessive physical labour

Excessive physical labour results in feebleness, emaciation, palpitations and dizziness.

Too little physical exercise causes a poor circulation, limp muscles, soft bones and obesity. This lowers the resistance of the body to disease.

Traumatic injuries

These are the same as in Western medicine.

Appendix

Stagnant blood and phlegm and humour are pathogenic products that may cause further pathological change if they are not eliminated. They have substantive and non-substantive meanings. Substantively they could be described as a blood clot or sputum, the non-substantive meaning is a generalization of a clinical syndrome, for instance, the stertorous breathing that may occur after a severe stroke is described as 'phlegm covering the orifice of the xin-heart'.

Stagnant blood
Stagnant blood can cause pain. The painful area is fixed and has a stabbing, boring or colicky nature.

Stagnant blood causes haemorrhage. This produces deep purple blood, often with clots.

Stagnant blood causes ecchymosis or petechia.

Stagnant blood can cause a mass. This can be any sort of mass, tumour, splenomegaly or hepatomegaly.

Phlegm and humour
Phlegm and humour are formed when water metabolism is disordered; an accumulation of excess water then turns into phlegm or humour. Phlegm and humour in the lung causes cough, dyspnoea and excessive sputum.

Phlegm and humour in the stomach causes abdominal distension and a succussion sound.

Phlegm covering the heart orifice causes coma and a rattling sound from the sputum in the throat, such as in a stroke.

Phlegm blocking the channels and collaterals causes hemiplegia, numbness of the extremities and difficulty in speech, such as in a stroke.

Phlegm accumulating subcutaneously occurs when there is a subcutaneous lymph node.

VI. DIFFERENTIATION OF DISEASE ACCORDING TO THE EIGHT PRINCIPLES

This is the diagnostic system of Chinese traditional medicine. The notes in the ensuing section explain the broad principles of diagnosis, using the history and examination of the patient as a basis.

Diseases are either *exterior* or *interior*. If a pathogen such as cold invades the body then it may be superficial or exterior in its damaging effect, such as the common cold, or it may be deep or interior, such as septicaemia. Usually diseases of the exterior show mild fever, headache, generalized aches and pains, and a superficial pulse. Diseases of the interior are characterized by a high fever, thirst, restlessness, delirium, vomiting, diarrhoea, a purplish-red tongue proper, with a white or yellow coating and a deep pulse.

Disease may be *hot* or *cold*. This means they may be due to the pathogen factors cold or heat. Diseases of heat show the signs of an acute infection or intestinal obstruction, whereas diseases of cold are more chronic in nature. Diseases of cold are characterized by a dislike of cold, pallor, loose stool, polyuria, a large flabby white tongue with a white coating, and a slow or deep and thready pulse. Diseases of heat show fever, dislike of heat, thirst, a red face, constipation, red scanty urine, and a red tongue proper with a yellow coating, associated with a rapid pulse.

Diseases may be *xu* or *shi*. Diseases of xu are usually more chronic in nature and are due to a deficiency of either the yin or the yang within the body. The patient is in low spirits, pale, emaciated, has palpitations and the tongue proper is light or red with a white or yellow coating, and there is a xu pulse. A shi disease is often more acute and is due to an excess of the yin or the yang within the body. This presents with irritability, distension and fullness of the chest and abdomen, scanty urine and dysuria, a red or white tongue proper with a yellow or white coating, and a shi or forceful pulse. There is a great deal of reference to xu and shi and it is important to realize that xu really means a deficiency, and shi really means an excess.

The last two principles are *yin* and *yang*. They are the generalization of the above ideas, which have already been discussed in Part I of this section.

VII. METHODS OF DIAGNOSIS

Inspection

Mental condition
See mental pathogens.

Facial complexion
A red face occurs with febrile diseases, a pale wizened face is due to anaemia or xu diseases, a yellow face occurs in jaundice and a purple face occurs in anoxia, severe pain or stagnation of blood.

Body build, posture and motion
In an obese person there is a chronic deficiency of qi with invasion of phlegm and damp, while in an emaciated person there is hyperactivity of fire due to a deficiency of yin. Paralysis of the limbs indicates insufficiency of qi and blood with blocked channels and collaterals. Convulsions and muscle spasm are often due to an invasion of the channels by wind, due to an insufficiency of yin.

Examination of the tongue
This is a most important diagnostic tool; the tongue is divided into the tongue proper and the tongue coating. A normal tongue has a pink tongue proper with a white clear coating over the tongue.

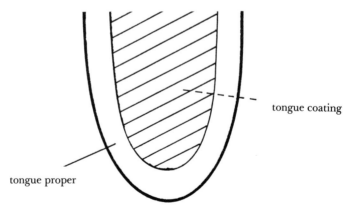

tongue coating

tongue proper

The Tongue.

The tongue proper

A light coloured tongue proper: A light tongue proper indicates insufficiency of qi and blood, invasion of cold, and xu of yang.

A red tongue proper: A red tongue proper indicates diseases due to heat, or internal diseases of heat due to xu of yin.

A purplish-red tongue proper: This occurs in acute diseases of heat when heat has been transmitted from the exterior of the body to the interior, for instance septicaemia. It can also be seen in diseases that exhaust the body fluid, causing hyperactivity of yang due to an insufficiency of yin, for instance terminal carcinoma.

A purplish tongue proper: A purple or bluish-purple tongue proper indicates retardation of qi and stagnation of blood, causing internal cold due to xu of yang, for instance ischaemic heart disease or heart failure.

A large flabby tongue proper: A large and flabby tongue proper with teeth marks indicates xu of qi and xu of yang, for instance chronic enteritis. If there are purplish-red spots on the tongue then this means that there is an invasion of heat.

A streaked tongue proper: Some people have a congenital streaked tongue (this is called a geographical tongue in Western medicine) and it must be ignored. Streaks or red prickles on the tongue normally indicate hyperactivity of fire causing consumption of the body fluid and this is often found after infectious diseases.

Stiff and tremulous tongue proper: The tongue shows fasci-culation and it may curl up. This is often accompanied by indistinct speech and mental disorders and indicates disturbance of the mind by phlegm and heat, or deficiency of yin of the gan-liver.

The tongue coating

A white coating: A thick white coating indicates stagnation of food, for instance dyspepsia.

A white greasy coating indicates invasion by the pathogen cold and damp, or phlegm, for instance chronic bronchitis.

A white powder-like coating indicates invasion by plague, for instance typhoid.

A yellow coating: A thick yellow coating indicates chronic indigestion.

A thin yellow coating indicates invasion of fei-lung by wind and heat, for instance a cold.

A greasy yellow coating indicates internal damp and heat, or phlegm and heat, for instance bacillary dysentery or a lung abscess.

A charring yellow coating indicates the accumulation of heat in the intestines which damages the yin, for instance infectious diseases of the intestine.

A yellow tongue coating may also be caused by smoking.

A greyish-black coating: A greyish-black slippery coating indicates excessive cold due to xu of yang, and this occurs in certain types of dyspepsia.

A greyish-black dry coating indicates exhaustion of the body fluids due to excessive heat, for instance dehydration.

A peeling coating: When the tongue coating is partially or completely peeled off the tongue proper can be seen. This indicates severe damage of the normal qi and an extreme deficiency of yin, for instance the late stages of terminal cancer.

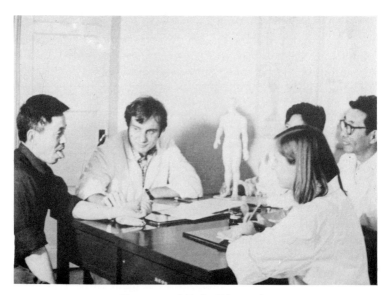

Tongue and Pulse Diagnosis.

Auscultation

Listening to the speech
Speaking in a low feeble voice indicates diseases of xu nature and sonorous speech indicates shi diseases. A partial loss of consciousness means that heat and phlegm are covering the heart orifice. Talking to oneself means that there is a derangement of the mind, and indistinct speech often means that the channels are blocked by wind and phlegm.

Listening to the respiration
Feeble respiration with dyspnoea and excessive sweating indicates xu of qi of the xin-heart and fei-lung. Heavy respiration, with a productive cough, indicates a shi disease of fei-lung due to an accumulation of phlegm and heat, or phlegm and humour, in fei-lung.

Listening to the cough
A heavy unclear cough is caused by invasion of fei-lung with wind and cold, or accumulation of cold and humour in fei-lung. A loud clear cough often indicates wind and heat, or phlegm and heat, in fei-lung. A dry cough with minimal sputum is often caused by a chronic xu of yin of fei-lung, for instance tuberculosis.

Smell
A rank foul smell of any discharge or secretion indicates a disease of shi nature (infection). A light smell indicates a disease of xu nature, for instance scanty red urine with a foul smell indicates a hot shi-disease, like cystitis, while clear profuse urine indicates a cold xu disease, like diabetes insipidus.

Interrogation
This is best summed up by the translation of an old Chinese text called the ten askings:

> One ask chill and fever, two perspiration, three ask head and trunk, four stool and urine, five food intake and six chest. Deafness and thirst are seven and eight, nine past history and ten causes. Besides this you should ask about the drugs taken, and for women patients you should ask their menstrual and obstetric history. Finally, for infants, ask about the normal childhood diseases.

This section is included purely for interest as the method of taking a history so clearly corresponds with that used in Western medicine.

Palpation

Palpation of the pulse

The pulse provides a great deal of the information gained from palpation, although a mass or trauma will obviously have to be examined on a more Westernized basis. In classical Chinese medicine there are six pulses at each wrist. These pulses occupy three positions at each wrist over the radial artery, and each position has a deep and superficial pulse. Each of these pulses represents a different organ and in this way all twelve of the zang fu organs are represented by a wrist pulse. The character of the pulse indicates the state of health of each organ and also the balance between each organ. Although traditional pulse diagnosis is still used in China we were taught a much simpler form of pulse 'generalization' rather than the traditional pulse diagnosis, and it is this pulse 'generalization' that will be discussed in the following section.

A superficial pulse: This pulse responds to the finger when pressed lightly and becomes weak on heavy pressure. It is often seen in the early stages of diseases caused by exogenous pathogens, such as infections.

A deep pulse: This pulse is not clear on superficial palpation but it is felt on deep pressure. It is often seen in interior diseases such as glomerulonephritis.

A slow pulse: This pulse is less than sixty beats per minute; it may be normal or it may be seen in atrio-venticular block, i.e. diseases of cold.

A rapid pulse: This pulse is greater than sixty beats per minute; it is often seen in diseases of heat.

A xu pulse: The pulse is weak and forceless and goes on heavy pressure. This is seen in diseases of xu nature, such as malnutrition or diseases of pi-spleen.

A shi pulse: The pulse is forceful and will not go on deep palpation; it is seen in shi diseases.

A large pulse: This is an abundant pulse; it is like a surging wave and is seen in diseases of shi nature and heat.

A thready pulse: This is like a thready flow of water and it is often seen in xu diseases.

A bowstring pulse: The pulse is hard and forceful and gives the sensation of pressing on the string of a bent bow. It may be normal or it may be seen in diseases where there is hyperactivity of the yang of the gan-liver.

A gliding pulse: This is round and forceful, like beads rolling on a plate. It is often seen in cases of indigestion or obstruction of phlegm. Sometimes a gliding pulse may be seen in a healthy person, especially in pregnancy.

An intermittent pulse: The pulse is irregular. This occurs in retardation of qi and stagnation of blood, causing a deficiency of qi in the xin-heart, such as atrial fibrillation.

Palpation for all other pathology, such as mass or trauma, follows the same rules as in Western medicine.

VIII. THE DIFFERENTIATION OF SYNDROMES

The Chinese described symptom pictures which allow the differentiation of specific Zang Fu syndromes. The major syndromes are described below and provide further useful information which will enable the acupuncturist to reach a clear Zang Fu diagnosis.

Syndromes of the Xin-heart

1. Weakness of the qi of the xin-heart
Clinical manifestations: Palpitations, dyspnoea aggravated by exertion, a pale tongue and a thready xu or irregular pulse. If there is evidence of a dificiency of the yang of the xin-heart then cold limbs, pallor, and purplish lips can be found. Exhaustion of the yang of the xin-heart may manifest itself as profuse sweating,

mental confusion and a fading, thready pulse.

Aetiology and pathology: This syndrome is usually caused by general malaise after anxiety or a long illness, which injures the qi of the xin-heart. When the qi of the xin-heart is weak it fails to pump blood normally resulting in palpitations, dyspnoea and a thready irregular or xu pulse. Alternatively, a prolonged weakness of the qi of the xin-heart may lead to weakness of the yang of the xin-heart. When the body lacks yang it lacks energy and heat, therefore symptoms such as chills, cold limbs and pallor occur. If the yang of the xin-heart is exhausted, the defensive qi of the body surface can no longer protect the essential qi and lets it dissipate, this results in profuse sweating and a fading, thready pulse.

2. Insufficiency of the yin of the xin-heart
Clinical manifestations: Palpitations, insomnia, dream-disturbed sleep, anxiety and possible malar flush with a low grade fever. A red tongue proper and a thready and rapid pulse will also be found.

Aetiology and pathology: This syndrome is usually due to damage of the yin by a febrile disease or anxiety, which consumes the yin of the xin-heart. Insufficiency of the yin of the xin-heart often leads to hyperactivity of the fibre of the xin-heart, resulting in the above symptoms. Insufficiency of the yin of the xin-heart may also cause insufficiency of the blood of the xin-heart. If this happens then there is not enough yin and blood to nourish the xin-heart, and the xin-heart fails in its function of keeping the mind. The symptoms of insomnia, poor memory and dream-disturbed sleep will therefore appear.

3. Stagnation of the blood of the heart
Clinical manifestations: Palpitations, cardiac retardation and pain (paroxysms of pricking pain, or in more severe cases colicky pain often referred to the shoulders and the back), peripheral and central cyanosis and a thready or irregular pulse.

Aetiology and pathology: This syndrome is due to anxiety leading to stagnation of qi and stagnation of blood. It may also be due to insufficiency of the qi of the xin-heart after a chronic illness; if the qi of the xin-heart is too weak to sustain the cardiac circulation then stagnation of blood of the xin-heart and obstruction of the blood vessels results. Stagnation of the blood often impedes the distribution of yang qi in the chest causing discomfort in the chest (angina) and peripheral cyanosis. A dark purplish tongue proper, or purple spots on the tongue, and a thready or irregular pulse are manifestations of stagnation of blood and confinement of the yang qi.

4. Hyperactivity of the fire of the xin-heart
Clinical manifestations: Ulceration, swelling and pain in the mouth and tongue, insomnia accompanied by fever, a flushed face, a bitter taste in the mouth, hot, dark and yellow urine, a red tongue proper and a rapid pulse.

Aetiology and pathology: This syndrome is often due to mental irritation which causes depression of qi. The depressed qi may turn into endogenous fire and disturb the mind, causing the symptoms of insomnia and fever to appear. As the xin-heart has the tongue as its orifice, and its function is reflected in the face, a disorder of the fire of the xin-heart may cause many of the above symptoms.

5. Derangement of the mind
Clinical manifestations: Depression, dullness, muttering to oneself, anxiety, incoherent speech, mania and in severe cases coma.

Aetiology and pathology: This syndrome is often due to mental irritation which causes depression of qi. The body fluid stagnates to form damp and/or phlegm which causes blurring of the xin-heart and mind, resulting in dullness and depression. If the depressed qi turns into fire and the phlegm and fire distrub the xin-heart, anxiety, incoherent speech and mania result. Blurring of the mind by phlegm and/or damp, or phlegm and/or fire causes coma. A high fever, coma and delirium resulting from invasion of the pericardium by heat, are due to pathogenic heat invading deep into the interior of the body and disturbing the mind.

Syndromes of the Gan-liver

1. Depression of the qi of the gan-liver

Clinical manifestations: Hypochondrial and lower-abdominal pain and distension, a distended sensation in the breasts, discomfort in the chest and belching, sighing, or a sensation of a foreign body in the throat. Women may experience irregular periods.

Aetiology and pathology: This syndrome is usually due to mental irritation causing depression of the qi of the gan-liver and stagnation of the qi in the liver channel. This leads to hypochondrial and lower abdominal pain and distension, a distended sensation in the breasts and discomfort in the chest. Stagnation of the qi of the gan-liver may affect the stomach, causing failure of the qi of the stomach to descend and resulting in belching. The sensation of a foreign body in the throat is due to stagnation of the qi of the liver channel, which with the phelgm forms a lump in the throat. Depression of the qi of the gan-liver and the subsequent lack of freeing may further impair the gan-liver's function of blood storage. Stagnation of qi leads to stagnation of blood, the cause of irregular periods.

2. Flare-up of the fire of the gan-liver

Clinical manifestations: Dizziness, a distended sensation in the head, headache, red eyes, a bitter taste in the mouth, a flushed face, irritability and sometimes haematemesis and epistaxis can occur. The tongue proper is red with a yellow coating and the pulse is wiry and rapid.

Aetiology and pathology: This syndrome is often due to a long-standing depression of the qi of the gan-liver which can turn into fire. It may also be due to over-indulgence in alcohol and tobacco causing an accumulation of heat which turns into fire. The upward disturbance of the fire of the gan-liver causes dizziness, a distended sensation in the head, headache, red eyes, a bitter taste in the mouth and a flushed face. Fire injures the gan-liver, causing impairment of its function in promoting the free flow of qi and this causes irritability. When the fire of the gan-liver injures the blood vessels it causes extravasation of blood and haematemesis and epistaxis can occur.

3. Stagnation of cold in the liver channel

Clinical manifestations: Lower-abdominal pain, swelling and distension in the testis with tenesmus. The scrotum may be cold and contracted and these symptoms can be alleviated by warmth. The tongue proper is pale with a white coating and the pulse deep and wiry or slow.

Aetiology and pathology: The liver channel curves around the external genitalia and passes through the lower abdomen. When cold, which is characterized by contraction and stagnation, stays in the liver channel, stagnation of the qi and blood may occur and cause lower-abdominal pain, swelling and distension of the testis with tenesmus. Cold and contraction of the scrotum are also due to the pathogen cold.

4. Insufficiency of the blood of the gan-liver

Clinical manifestations: Dizziness, blurred vision, dry eyes, pallor, spasm of the tendons and muscles, numb limbs and a scanty light-coloured menstrual flow with a prolonged cycle.

Aetiology and pathology: This syndrome often occurs after a haemorrhage or another chronic disease in which blood is destroyed, and the reserves of the gan-liver are depleted, thereby resulting in a failure of the gan-liver to nourish the channels. A xu (deficiency) of blood may cause endogenous wind so that the symptoms of muscle spasticity and numb limbs appear. An upward disturbance of endogenous wind (xu type) can cause dizziness and blurred vision. Insufficiency of the blood of the gan-liver and disruption of its blood storage function results in emptiness of the chong channel which will cause menstrual abnormalities.

5. Stirring of the wind of the gan-liver by heat

Clinical manifestations: High fever, convulsions, neck rigidity (opisthotonos) and coma. A deep-red tongue proper and a wiry, rapid pulse are also found.

Aetiology and pathology: This syndrome is due to transmission of the pathogen heat from the exterior to the interior, which burns the yin of the gan-liver and deprives the tendons and blood vessels of nourishment. Furthermore, pathogenic heat in the interior stirs up endogenous wind causing fever, convulsions and neck rigidity. Coma is due to pathogenic heat affecting the pericardium and disturbing the mind.

Syndromes of the Pi-spleen

1. Weakness of the qi of the pi-spleen
Clinical manifestations: Sallow complexion, anorexia, loose stools, oedema, and lassitude. There may be distension and a bearing-down sensation in the abdomen, a prolapse of the rectum and/or uterus, or a chronic blood disorder such as purpura, bloody stools or uterine bleeding. A pale tongue proper and a thready xu pulse will be found on examination. If there is evidence of xu (deficiency) of the yang of the pi-spleen, symptoms of cold such as cold limbs will occur.

Aetiology and pathology: This syndrome is often caused by irregular food intake, excessive mental strain or chronic disease. These problems result in weakness of the qi of the pi-spleen and impair its function of transportation and transformation, which consequently results in a poor appetite and loose stools. Accumulation of fluid in the interior is the cause of the oedema. The general malaise is due to a lack of food failing to provide a nourishing basis for blood formation. When the qi of the pi-spleen is weak, it loses its ability to uplift tissues so that there is distension, a bearing-down sensation in the abdomen and a prolapse of the rectum and/or uterus. Weakness of the qi of the pi-spleen also causes the blood disorders. Xu (deficiency) of the yan of the pi-spleen causes cold limbs.

2. Invasion of the pi-spleen by cold and damp
Clinical manifestations: Fullness and distension in the chest and epigastrium, a poor appetite, a heavy feeling in the head, malaise, borborygmii, abdominal pain and loose stools. A white sticky tongue coating and a thready pulse will be found.

Aetiology and pathology: This syndrome usually occurs after rain, or it may be due to over-indulgence of raw or cold food. In both cases the pathogen cold and damp injurs the pi-spleen impairing its function of transportation and transformation and resulting in a poor appetite, borborygmii, abdominal pain and loose stools. As pathogenic damp is sticky and stagnant, it is liable to block the flow of qi causing a sensation of epigastric fullness and distension.

Syndromes of the fei-lung

1. Invasion of the fei-lung by the pathogen wind
Clinical manifestations: An itchy throat and cough associated with fever and chills. If the wind is accompanied by cold then the patient usually feels cold and presents with nasal obstruction, a watery nasal discharge and mucoid sputum. The tongue coating is thin and white. If the wind is associated with heat, fever will be the most prominent symptom and will be associated with a red, swollen throat, a purulent nasal discharge and purulent sputum. The tongue coating will be yellow.

Aetiology and pathology: Invasion of the fei-lung by the pathogen wind disturbs its function of dispersal and descent. Normal respiration is affected producing the symptoms of cough and nasal obstruction. Cold is a yin pathogen and therefore liable to damage the yang qi. Consequently when wind is associated with cold, the sensation of cold will be more severe than that of fever and will be accompanied by a watery nasal discharge and white mucoid sputum. Heat is a yang pathogen, and if wind is accompanied by heat, fever will become the most prominent symptom and will be associated with a purulent nasal discharge and purulent sputum.

2. Retention of damp and/or phlegm in the fei-lung
Clinical manifestations: Cough, dyspnoea and white frothy sputum. The onset is generally precipitated by cold, and the tongue coating is white and sometimes sticky.

Aetiology and pathology: This syndrome is due to the disturbance of the normal circulation of body fluid, the body fluid accumulates and precipitates the formation of damp/or phlegm. When damp and phlegm remain in the fei-lung the passage of qi is blocked and the functions of the fei-lung are impaired, this results in the above symptoms.

3. Retention of phlegm and/or heat in the fei-lung

Clinical manifestations: Cough, dyspnoea, wheezing and thick yellow and/or green sputum (occasionally pus). This can be associated with rigors and a fever; the tongue proper is red with a yellow coating and there is a rapid pulse.

Aetiology and pathology: This syndrome is caused by invasion of exogenous wind and/or heat, or wind and/or cold, which later develops into heat. The heat mixes with phlegm, which remains in the fei-lung and blocks the circulation of qi; this impairs the functions of the fei-lung and causes cough, dyspnoea and wheeze. Heat exhausts body fluid causing purulent sputum. When phlegm and heat are found in the fei-lung, stagnation of blood results which in turn leads to purulent, bloody sputum.

4. Insufficiency of the yin of the fei-lung

Clinical manifestations: A dry, unproductive cough associated with sticky, scant, blood-stained sputum, fever, a malar flush, a feverish sensation in the palms and soles, a dry mouth and night sweats. A red tongue proper and a thready and rapid pulse will be found.

Aetiology and pathology: Such symptoms are usually caused by chronic disease of the fei-lung, which consumes the yin and results in insufficiency of body fluid. The fei-lung is deprived of nourishment, its functions are impaired and this produces a dry mouth. Xu (deficiency) of yin causes endogenous heat which drives out body fluid and injures blood vessels, this results in a fever, a malar flush, a feverish sensation in the palms and soles, night sweats and bloody sputum.

Syndromes of the Shen-kidney

1. Weakness of the qi of the shen-kidney

Clinical manifestations: A sore and weak sensation in the lumbar region and knee joints, urinary frequency, polyuria, dribbling, enuresis, urinary incontinence, dyspnoea, wheezing, and occasionally infertility. The pulse will be thready.

Aetiology and pathology: This syndrome is often caused by

malaise after a prolonged chronic illness, or may be the result of senility or congenital deficiency. Weakness of the qi of the shen-kidney results in an inability of the urinary bladder to control urination; this causes enuresis, incontinence, frequency and urgency. Shen-kidney stores essence (shen), but when the qi of the shen-kidney is deficient, infertility can result. When the qi of the shen-kidney is weak, it fails to help the fei-lung perform its function of descent, qi therefore attacks the fei-lung resulting in dyspnoea and wheezing.

2. Insufficiency of the yang of the shen-kidney
Clinical manifestations: These are broadly similar to the syndrome described as 'Weakness of qi of the shen-kidney'. The major symptoms are a dull ache in the lumbar region and knee joints, cold, pallor, impotence, oliguria and oedema of the lower limbs. A pale, tooth-marked tongue and a deep thready pulse will be found.

Aetiology and pathology: This syndrome usually occurs after a prolonged chronic illness in which the yang of the shen-kidney is injured, it may occasionally be due to an excess of sexual activity which also injures the yang of the shen-kidney. In either instance, the yang of the shen-kidney fails to warm the body which results in cold aching sensations in the low back and knee joints, and impotence. Then shen-kidney controls water metabolism, and an insufficiency of the yang of the shen-kidney results in oliguria; the subsequent fluid excess presents with the symptom of oedema.

3. Insufficiency of the yin of the shen-kidney
Clinical manifestations: Blurred vision, tinnitus, amnesia, feverish sensation in the palms and soles, a malar flush, night sweats, hot yellow urine and constipation. The tongue proper will be red and the pulse thready and rapid.

Aetiology and pathology: This usually occurs after a prolonged chronic illness in which the yin of the shen-kidney is impaired, it may also be due to an over-indulgence in sexual activity, which consumes the shen-kidney. Either of these factors can result in the shen-kidney failing to produce marrow and maintaining normal cerebral function. The symptoms that result are dizziness, blurred vision, amnesia and tinnitus. A deficiency of the yin causes endogenous heat, which in turn consumes body fluid; this results in a feverish sensation in the palms and soles, a malar flush, night sweats, hot yellow urine and constipation.

Syndromes of the Pericardium
The syndromes of the pericardium are seen clinically as the invasion of the pericardium by heat. The symptoms are a high fever, coma and delirium, these result from heat invading the interior of the body, which in turn disturbs the mind.

Syndromes of the Small Intestine
Disturbance of the function of the small intestine is included in the syndromes of the pi-spleen, particularly with respect to its main function (transformation and transportation).

Syndromes of the Gall Bladder

Damp and heat in the gall bladder
Clinical manifestations: Yellow sclera and skin, pain in the costal and hypochondrial region, pain in the right upper abdominal quadrant and a bitter taste in the mouth. Some patients may vomit sour and/or bitter fluid. The tongue coating is yellow and sticky.

Aetiology and pathology: The function of the gall bladder is to store and excrete bile, and this depends on the normal function of the gan-liver. Exogenous damp and/or heat (heat caused by depression of the gan-liver, damp and heat caused by over-indulgence in alcohol and rich food) may accumulate in the gan-liver and gall bladder, thereby impairing the free flow of qi. Bile cannot therefore be secreted and freely excreted, and the subsequent biliary overflow causes jaundice, a bitter taste in the mouth and vomiting. Stagnation of the qi of the gan-liver and gall bladder also leads to stagnation of blood, causing right hypochondrial pain. This syndrome is closely related to the gan-liver, and is also known as 'damp and heat in the gan-liver and gall bladder'.

Syndromes of the Stomach

1. Retention of food in the stomach
Clinical manifestations: Distension and pain in the epigastric region, anorexia, belching, heartburn and vomiting. The tongue has a thick sticky coating.

Aetiology and pathology: This syndrome is usually caused by over-eating, which leads to the retention of undigested food in the stomach; the qi of the stomach ascends rather than descending.

2. Retention of fluid in the stomach due to cold
Clinical manifestations: The sensation of fullness associated with a dull epigastric pain, aggravated by cold and alleviated by warmth. The tongue coating will be white and sticky and the pulse thready or slow.

Aetiology and pathology: This syndrome usually follows a cold after rain, or may be precipitated by the excessive ingestion of raw or cold food. Either of these factors result in cold in the stomach which causes stagnation of qi and pain. Prolonged damage injures the yang qi of the pi-spleen and stomach so that body fluid is retained in the stomach instead of being transported and transformed, this results in vomiting.

3. Hyperactivity of the fire of the stomach
Clinical manifestations: A burning in the epigastrium, thirst, a preference for cold drinks, vomiting of undigested food or sour fluid, gingival swelling pain and ulceration, halitosis. The tongue proper will be red with a dry yellow coating.

Aetiology and pathology: This syndrome is usually due to over-eating rich food, which causes heat to accumulate in the stomach. The heat consumes body fluid and causes the qi of the stomach to ascend. This results in a burning epigastric pain, thirst, a preference for cold drinks and vomiting. Halitosis and gingival ulceration are due to the fire element in the stomach.

Syndromes of the Large Intestine

1. Damp and heat in the large intestine
Clinical manifestations: Fever, abdominal pain, loose dark smelly stools, frequent bowel movements. White or red mucus may be present in the stool, and can be associated with perineal pain and tenesmus. The tongue proper is red with a yellow coating, and the pulse rolling and rapid.

Aetiology and pathology: This syndrome is usually caused by eating too much raw, cold or contaminated food. It may also be due to invasion of summer heat and damp. Damp and heat accumulate in the large intestine, blocking the passage of qi and disturbing its function of transmission and transformation; this produces diarrhoea, abdominal pain and dark smelly stool. Damp and heat may also injure the blood vessels of the large intestine producing bloody mucus in the stool. The downward pressure of the damp and heat causes perineal pain and tenesmus.

2. Stasis of the large intestine
Clinical manifestations: A distended full abdomen, abdominal pain (intensified with pressure), constipation, nausea and vomiting. The tongue coating is white and sticky and the pulse shi and deep.

Aetiology and pathology: This syndrome may be due to food retention, gastro-intestinal parasites, or blood stagnation; all these factors cause obstruction of the qi and functional derangement of the large intestine. This results in constipation, abdominal distension and pain. The nausea and vomiting are caused by the qi of the large intestine impeding the descending qi of the stomach.

3. Stagnation of blood and heat in the large intestine
Clinical manifestations: A severe boring or fixed pain in the lower abdomen, which is made worse by pressure, constipation and/or mild diarrhoea, fever and vomiting. The tongue proper is red with a yellow sticky coating.

Aetiology and pathology: This syndrome is usually due to the individual's failure to adapt to changes in the weather, or may be caused by over-eating and/or excessive exercise. These factors result in stagnation of heat and blood and retardation of qi; heat injures the vessels of the large intestine, causing local inflammation and pain in the lower abdomen. If the qi of the stomach is affected then this can result in nausea and vomiting.

Syndromes of the Urinary Bladder

1. Damp and heat in the urinary bladder
Clinical manifestations: Frequency, urgency, dysuria, blood-stained urine and the presence of clots or stones in the urine. The tongue proper will be red with a yellow coating, and the pulse rapid.

Aetiology and pathology: Damp and heat injures the urinary bladder and disturbs its function of storing urine, this results in frequency and urgency. When damp and heat injure the blood vessels of the urinary bladder, stagnation of blood and heat occur leading to haematuria and blood clots in the urine. Prolonged retention of damp and heat in the bladder results in stone formation.

2. Disturbance in the function of the urinary bladder
Clinical manifestations: Dribbling, weak stream, urinary retention, a lumbar ache associated with pain in the knee joints and a dislike of cold. The tongue proper is pale with a white coating, and the pulse thready and deep (xu).

Aetiology and pathology: This syndrome is due to an insufficiency of the yang of the shen-kidney and impairment of its function of urinary filtration. The symptoms of cold therefore result, such as a dislike of cold, cold extremities and weakness and pain in the lumbar region and knee joints.

Syndromes of the Sanjiao
The syndromes of the sanjiao relate to the organs present in the upper, middle and lower jiao. Obstruction of the upper jiao usually refers to confinement of the qi of the fei-lung, insufficiency of the qi of the middle jiao refers to weakness of the pi-

spleen and stomach and damp and heat in the lower jiao refers to damp and heat in the urinary bladder. The Sanjiao cannot be explained as a single entity.

IX. CONCLUSION

The principles that are outlined in this section enable the acupuncturist to use traditional medicine to find out which organ is diseased, and what pathogen is causing that disease. This allows the classical differentiation of syndromes, and the subsequent determination of treatment based on the differentiation of the symptoms and signs. In essence this represents a simplified form of the pure traditional Chinese medicine. It is a fairly swift method to understand and it is also accurate. Because there are so many different concepts to absorb it is very difficult to explain each one as it occurs in the text, but ultimately the text fits together as a system. We therefore suggest that the reader goes through it initially without trying to understand it all at once; it should be much clearer on a second reading.

Furthermore, we wish to stress that this information will only tell the acupuncturist what the problem is. Point selection, and the rules that govern this, are discussed in the next section, but it is essential to understand this initial theory before the rules of point selection will make sense.

THE PRINCIPLES OF THERAPY

In the first section we discussed the principles of Chinese medicine which will enable a traditional diagnosis to be made. This knowledge provides a basis for treatment.

I. THE PRINCIPLES OF DISEASE

Diseases fall into two main groups, diseases of the channels and collaterals, and diseases of the zang and fu organs.

Diseases of the Channels and Collaterals
These are the diseases of the superficial channels of the body — arthritis and acute strains are examples of this type of disease. The internal yin and yang balance is normal but the flow of qi and blood through the channels is disrupted. This usually presents with pain and is called a disease of 'bi' or blockage of the channels. If the flow of qi and blood is restored then the pain will go. This is the main therapeutic principle that is applied for this type of disease.

Diseases of the Zang and Fu Organs
These are the diseases of the internal organs of the body where there is an imbalance of the yin and yang within the body. Neurasthenia and asthma are clear examples of this type of disease. To treat these problems it is essential to be able to make a

clear traditional diagnosis and to know the rules of point selection.

Diseases that Combine Zang and Fu, and Channel Disorders

A disease of pain, such as migraine, may combine these two ideas. Migraine is usually a disorder of the gan-liver but there is also a blockage of the flow of qi and blood in the channels around the temple, resulting in pain. The channels and collaterals, and the zang fu, will therefore both require treatment in this disease.

II. PRINCIPLES OF POINT SELECTION

Diseases of the Channels and Collaterals

The principle of treatment for these diseases is to select the local points (Ah shi points or acupuncture points), and also a distal point on the channel that crosses the painful area. The local painful points are quite simple to find when the patient is examined, but the distal points are a matter of experience. There are no rules for the selection of these distal points, they have just been handed on to us as a product of empirical experience.

Local points

The local points are outlined in the discussion on each disease. There are common painful points in each type of disease and these are included in the prescriptions. The disease may not be typical, and the local points may vary a little, so do not follow the prescription blindly but examine the painful area and use the points that seem most relevant. The tender point, or the Ah shi point (both mean the same thing) also has a part to play in this type of disease. If you find a very tender area that does not seem to be an acupuncture point then use it as well as the local acupuncture points. The tender point is often an acupuncture point that you have not learnt.

Distal points

These are part of the basic grammar of acupuncture and they just have to be learnt. The easiest way to do this is to give a list of the most important distal points, with their uses.

Houxi (SI 3) This point may be used for pain over the small intestine channel, especially pain from cervical syndrome that is referred to the scapular area.

Hegu (LI 4) This point may be used for pain over the large intestine channel and it is also a very important point for facial pain, headache and sinusitis.

Quchi (LI 11) This is often used as a distal point for referred pain from the shoulder or neck.

Waiguan (SJ 5) This is the most important distal point in the upper limb. If there is pain in the upper limb that is not on a channel then this point may be used. It is also used when there is pain over the Sanjiao channel.

Weizhong (UB 40) This point is used for low back pain, or any pain over the lower part of the urinary bladder channel.

Kunlun (UB 60) This point is used for upper thoracic, cervical pain or headache, i.e. pain over the upper part of the urinary bladder channel.

Yanglingquan (GB 34) This may be used for any pain over the gall bladder channel, such as migraine.

Neiting (St 44) This is used for pain over the stomach channel such as facial pain, abdominal pain or hip pain radiating down the front of the leg.

These are the most important distal points. For some diseases of 'bi' no distal points are used, and the common diseases where these exceptions apply are knee pain, ankle pain, wrist pain, hand pain and foot pain. In these diseases use only the local points as outlined in the prescriptions. Sometimes the local acupuncture points may not be tender until they are carefully examined.

Diseases of the Zang and Fu Organs
On the basis of traditional diagnosis the acupuncturist will be able to decide what organ is diseased and what pathogen is causing that disease. He will then know which channel to use to correct the problem, and whether to sedate or tonify a particular organ. He must also dispel the pathogen, for instance, in cases of cold, he will need to warm with moxa or cupping or both.

There are many different rules that can be applied in order to select a point for a particular disease, but an experienced acupuncturist will often select only a few points. Initially this will be very confusing to a beginner, but as more clinical experience is obtained then it will slowly become clear that experience is the basis of many prescriptions. There are no dogmatic rules governing point selection for the zang fu diseases but there are several groups of special points that represent each organ. The most therapeutically useful groups are discussed and listed.

Back shu and front mu points

These points represent the surface points of the organs, the mu points are on the front and the shu points are on the back. If the zang organs are diseased (yin organs) then the back shu points are particularly effective, and if the fu organs are diseased (yang organs) then the front mu points are useful.

The shu points can be alternated with points on the ventral surface of the body, as outlined in some of the prescriptions. The back shu points are particularly useful in treating a zang disorder when it is associated with back pain, primarily because the position of the patient for acupuncture is much simpler.

TABLE I

Organ	Back Shu point	Front Mu point
Lung	Feishu (UB 13)	Zhongfu (Lu 1)
Pericardium	Jueyinshu (UB 14)	Shanzhong (Ren 17)
Heart	Xinshu (UB 15)	Jujue (Ren 14)
Liver	Ganshu (UB 18)	Qimen (Liv 14)
Gall bladder	Danshu (UB 19)	Riyue (GB 24)
Spleen	Pishu (UB 20)	Zhangmen (Liv 13)
Stomach	Weishu (UB 21)	Zhongwan (Ren 12)
Sanjiao	Sanjiaoshu (UB 22)	Shimen (Ren 5)
Kidney	Shenshu (UB 23)	Jingmen (GB 25)
Large intestine	Dachangshu (UB 25)	Tianshu (St 25)
Small intestine	Xiaochangshu (UB 27)	Guanyuan (Ren 4)
Urinary bladder	Pangguangshu (UB 28)	Zhongji (Ren 3)

The back shu points are prefixed by the Chinese name for the organ, for instance pi means spleen and pishu is the back shu point for the spleen; wei means stomach and weishu is the back shu point for the stomach.

Yuan source points
These points are near the wrist and the ankle. They are very useful points for treating diseases of their respective organs, for instance Taixi (K 3) and Taichong (Liv 3) are points commonly used for diseases of the gan-liver and shen-kidney; both are yuan source points. See Table II.

Luo connecting points
Each channel is connected internally and externally with another channel; for instance the lung and large intestine channels are connected. The luo connecting point is the actual connection

between these two channels, so the diseases of the connected channel can be treated by using the luo connecting point; for instance disease of the large intestine channel may be treated by using Lieque (Lu 7).

TABLE II

Channel	Yuan point	Luo point
Lung channel	Taiyuan (Lu 9)	Pianli (LI 6)
Large intestine channel	Hegu (LI 4)	Lieque (Lu 7)
Stomach channel	Chongyang (St 42)	Gongsun (Sp 4)
Spleen channel	Taibai (Sp 3)	Fenglong (St 40)
Heart channel	Shenmen (H 7)	Zhizheng (SI 7)
Small intestine channel	Hand-Wangu (SI 4)	Tongli (H 5)
Urinary bladder channel	Jinggu (UB 64)	Dazhong (K 4)
Kidney channel	Taixi (K 3)	Feiyang (UB 58)
Pericardium channel	Daling (P 7)	Waiguan (SJ 5)
Sanjiao channel	Yangchi (SJ 4)	Neiguan (P 6)
Gall bladder channel	Qiuxu (GB 40)	Ligou (Liv 5)
Liver channel	Taichong (Liv 3)	Guangming (GB 37)

Influential points

These points are often used when a disease relates to a specific tissue or organ. Zhongwan (Ren 12) is often used when there is abdominal pain because it is the influential point for the fu organs.

TABLE III

Tissues	The influential point
Zang organs	Zhangmen (Liv 13)
Fu organs	Zhongwan (Ren 12)
Qi (respiratory system)	Shanzhong (Ren 17)
Blood	Geshu (UB 17)
Tendon	Yanglingquan (GB 34)
Bone	Dazhu (UB 11)
Marrow	Xuanzhong (GB 39)
Arterial pulse	Taiyuan (Lu 9)

There are other groups of points, such as the Xi-cleft points or the lower He points, but they are of limited clinical value. The most important and frequently used groups of points have been mentioned.

The law of the five elements
No acupuncture book is complete without this, although we did not make a great deal of use of this law in our course.

There are five elements in traditional Chinese philosophy: wood, fire, earth, metal and water. Wood is represented by the liver and gall bladder, water the kidney and urinary bladder, fire the heart and small intestine, earth the spleen and stomach, and metal the lung and large intestine. There is a creating and destroying cycle for these elements.

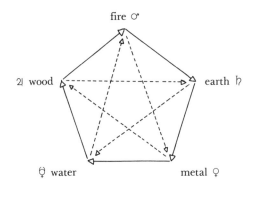

creating
destroying

The Law of the Five Elements.

TABLE IV(a)

Five Shu Points		Pt. Shu I Metal	Pt. Shu II Water	Pt. Shu III Wood	Pt. Shu IV Fire	Pt. Shu V Earth
Large Intestine	Metal	Shang-yang (LI 1)	Erijan (LI 2)	Sanjian (LI 3)	Yangxi (LI 5)	Quchi (LI 11)
Sanjiao	Fire	Guan-chong (SJ 1)	Yemen (SJ 2)	Zhongzhu (SJ 3)	Zhigou (SJ 6)	Tianjing (SJ 10)
Small Intestine	Fire	Shaoze (SI 1)	Qiangu (SI 2)	Houxi (SI 3)	Yanggu (SI 5)	Xiaohai (SI 8)
Stomach	Earth	Lidui (St 45)	Neiting (St 44)	Xiangu (St 43)	Jiexi (St 41)	Zusanli (St 36)
Gall Bladder	Wood	Foot-Qiaoyin (GB 44)	Xiaxi (GB 43)	Foot-Linqi (GB 41)	Yangfu (GB 38)	Yang-lingquan (GB 34)
Urinary Bladder	Water	Zhiyin (UB 67)	Tonggu (UB 66)	Shugu (UB 65)	Kunlun (UB 60)	Weizhong (UB 40)

TABLE IV(b)

Five Shu Points	Pt.Shu I Jing-Well Wood	Pt.Shu II Yung-Spring Fire	Pt.Shu III Shu-Stream Earth	Pt.Shu IV Jing-River Metal	Pt.Shu V He-Sea Water
Lung Metal	Shaoshang (Lu 11)	Yuji (Lu 10)	Taiyuan (Lu 9)	Jingqu (Lu 8)	Chize (Lu 5)
Pericardium Fire	Zhong-chong (P 9)	Laogong (P 8)	Daling (P 7)	Jianshi (P 5)	Quze (P 3)
Heart Fire	Shao-chong (H 9)	Shaofu (H 8)	Shenmen (H 7)	Lingdao (H 4)	Shaohai (H 3)
Spleen Earth	Yinbai (Sp 1)	Dadu (Sp 2)	Taibai (Sp 3)	Shangqiu (Sp 5)	Ying-lingquan (Sp 9)
Liver Wood	Dadun (Liv 1)	Xingjian (Liv 2)	Taichong (Liv 3)	Zhongfeng (Liv 4)	Ququan (Liv 8)
Kidney Water	Yongquan (K 1)	Rangu (K 2)	Taixi (K 3)	Fuliu (K 7)	Yingu (K 10)

Each channel has a point on it that represents each of the five elements. For the zang organs the jing-well points are wood, the yung-spring points are fire, the shu-stream points are earth, the jing-river points are metal and the he-sea points are water. For the fu organs jing-well is metal, yung-spring is water, shu-stream is wood, jing-river is fire and he-sea is earth.

These points, and the system they entail, may be used to tonify or sedate an organ. Wood creates fire, so fire is the 'son' of wood and wood is the 'mother' of fire. If the organ has a xu disease then the 'mother' point is used to tonify the diseased organ, for instance, if there is xu of xin-heart (fire) then use the mother point (wood) to tonify the heart. The wood point on the heart channel is Shaochong (H 9). If there is a shi disease of the xin-heart (fire) use the 'son' point (earth) to sedate the xin-heart. The earth point on the heart channel is Shenmen (H 7). Shenmen (H 7) is nearly always used for diseases of the xin-heart because most diseases of the xin-heart are shi in nature.

This law is explained at great length in many other texts, and the foregoing gives you a basic idea of what it entails. This, in fact, is the extent to which it was touched on in the course we attended.

Points according to symptoms

In diseases of the zang and fu organs there are many points that can be used for symptoms such as nausea. There are also some very useful points that can be used to dispel various pathogens. In this section we list some of the more useful points:

Taiyuan (Lu 9) can be used for cough, haematemasis and nasal obstruction.

Neiguan (P 6) can be used for palpitations, nausea, vomiting and insomnia.

Shenmen (H 7) can be used for palpitations, insomnia and diseases of the xin-heart.

Hegu (LI 4) can be used for fever, rhinitis, facial nerve paralysis and the dispersal of wind.

Waiguan (SJ 5) can be used for colds, fever, headache and strained neck.

Houxi (SI 3) can be used for tinnitus and malaria.

Sanyinjiao (Sp 6) can be used for disorders of the pi-spleen, impotence, irregular menstruation, enuresis, dysuria and insomnia.

Taichong (Liv 3) can be used for headaches, vertigo, eye diseases, pain in the costal and hypochondriac region, insomnia and diseases of the gan-liver.

Taixi (K 3) can be used for enuresis, dysuria, inspiratory dyspnoea, tinnitus, tooth cavities, chronic diarrhoea, poor vision, vertigo and impotence. This is an important point in deficiency diseases and diseases of the shen-kidney.

Zusanli (St 36) can be used for diseases of pi-spleen and general tonification.

Baihui (Du 20) can be used for headaches, dizziness, lifting (in vaginal or rectal prolapse), and mental diseases.

Quchi (LI 11) can be used for dispersing wind and heat.

Fenglong (St 40) can be used for resolving damp and phlegm.

Dazhui (Du 14) can be used for resolving fever and malaria.

Shanzhong (Ren 17) can be used for asthma, bronchitis and hiccoughs.

Zhongwan (Ren 12) can be used for disorders of the fu organs, such as vomiting or abdominal pain.

Guanyuan (Ren 4) can be used for general tonification, diseases of xu, enuresis and impotence.

Qihai (Ren 6) can be used as a point of general tonification.

Yintang (Extra) can be used for insomnia and neurasthenia.

A combination of the rules of point selection, as well as selecting the points according to the symptoms, has been used to make up the prescriptions in the following sections. Many of the points that are listed as points according to symptoms have complex traditional reasons behind their selection. They have been shown to be useful points by using a combination of traditional medicine and Chinese experience. The choice of prescription for a particular disease is not always easy and experience may be the most important factor in making that choice.

III. THE TENDER OR AH SHI POINT

The tender point is called the Ah shi point by the Chinese. A tender point(s) is often found in painful diseases and the acupuncturist will be guided to this point(s) by and through clinical examination and experience. In many cases the Ah shi point(s) may be felt as a pea-sized nodule(s) under the skin, or the patient may draw the attention of the acupuncturist to a painful area.

The Ah shi point(s) should always be used, especially in diseases of pain, along with local acupuncture points. In some cases they may replace the use of the acupuncture points as none of the acupuncture points will be near the affected area, or none of them may be tender.

The Ah shi point(s) should be treated as an acupuncture

point(s) and used as part of a normal prescription with other local and distal points. The acupuncturist must also remember that the Ah shi point(s) will often change from treatment to treatment and the patient should be examined thoroughly on each occasion.

IV. STIMULATION OF ACUPUNCTURE POINTS

Acupuncture is not the only way to stimulate an acupuncture point. Classical traditional medicine also involves the use of cupping and moxa to stimulate the points, and in some diseases these methods are preferable to using a needle. Certain points are impracticable for cupping, such as points on the arm and leg, and other points are forbidden to moxa, such as Jingming (UB 1).

When the needle is inserted the acupuncturist must be aware of the underlying tissues and organs. When a needle is being used on a point that is over the lung it must be inserted obliquely to avoid the danger of a pneumothorax. Common sense and a knowledge of basic anatomy should avoid any untoward accidents. The needle must also be sterilized properly so that there is no possibility of transmitting serum hepatitis.

It is important to remember that the piece of skin into which you insert the needle is relatively unimportant as long as the needle stimulates the acupuncture point. The needle for Shenmen (H 7) can be inserted in several different ways but the acupuncture point has been stimulated only if the needling sensation is felt. The actual acupuncture point is always underneath the skin, and it may be an inch or more deep to the dermis. The best method of knowing that you have stimulated an acupuncture point is to obtain deqi over that point. This means that the tip of the needle is the best point locator that the acupuncturist has at his disposal.

Stimulation of the Needle

Deqi
Deqi means needling sensation. This sensation is difficult to describe unless you have actually felt it; it is not pleasant though it is not painful. Deqi is slightly different for each point. Points on the head usually have a burning or pricking sensation, whereas

points on the limbs usually have a bursting, sore, full or numb sensation when they are stimulated. The needling sensation can travel up or down the channel.

The needle is stimulated by a perpendicular and rotary movement, lifting and thrusting the needle whilst it is being rotated. The only way to become competent at obtaining deqi is to practise.

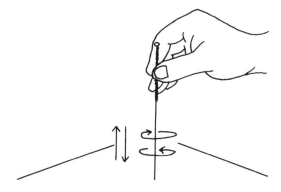

lifting and thrusting   rotation

Manipulating an Acupuncture Needle.

Unless the acupuncturist obtains deqi over each acupuncture point used then the acupuncture point has not been stimulated, and this means that the acupuncture is of questionable value.

Electrical stimulation
It is impossible to be dogmatic about the use of electrical stimulation as so much work is being done in this area at the moment. The Chinese are not the best people to give a clear picture of the use of stimulators. In general the stimulator is used in anaesthesia and when it is used therapeutically it is used for conditions of severe pain, acute conditions, scalp acupuncture, and conditions where ordinary needling has failed. The Chinese do not use it very much for treating disease.

Manual stimulation
The reducing method is used in acute or shi diseases, and the reinforcing method is used in chronic or xu diseases. Strong

stimulation is approximately equivalent to the reducing method and weak stimulation is roughly equivalent to the reinforcing method. This is all dependent on the individual as strong stimulation of a sensitive patient may be equivalent to weak stimulation of a less sensitive person. In weak stimulation the manipulation of the needle should be stopped as soon as the patient feels deqi, in strong stimulation the needle should be stimulated until the needling sensation is intense.

Reactions
If a patient is overstimulated then this may cause a temporary worsening of the condition. This is transitory and indicates a response to acupuncture. If this occurs then stimulate less forcefully next time.

Patients receiving acupuncture for the first time
Because of the possibility of a reaction stimulate the needles gently on the first visit. Needles are usually inserted proximally first, but in those receiving treatment for the first time it is less distressing to use the distal points first.

Moxibustion and Cupping
Both moxibustion and cupping are methods of stimulating an acupuncture point. They are nearly always used in diseases of cold where the main treatment is to warm the affected area. The indications for moxa and cupping are mentioned in the treatment of each specific disease, but in general cupping is usually the preferred method of warming a point, and where this is impracticable, such as on a limb or on the face, moxa is used.

Moxa is made from the dried leaves of Artemesia Vulgaris, and the older the moxa the more effective it is. Moxa can be used in several different forms. Loose moxa, or moxa punk, can be made into small cones and burnt on the skin (it is removed before it burns) or it may be burnt on a slice of ginger or garlic.

Moxa sticks may also be used. These are rolls of moxa which can be used to heat the skin directly, or they can be cut and burnt on the end of a needle. This method of warm handling allows heat to travel directly into the acupuncture point.

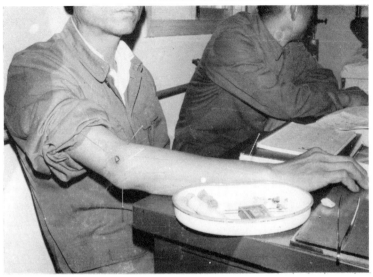

Moxa Cone for the Treatment of Tennis Elbow.

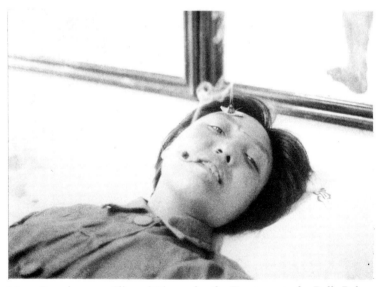

Moxa Burning on a Slice of Ginger for the Treatment of a Bells Palsy.

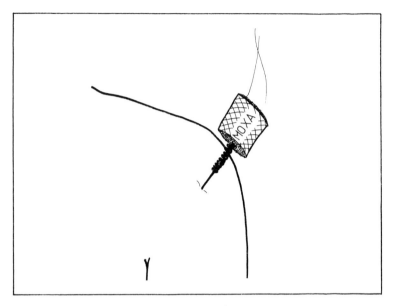

Warm Needling.

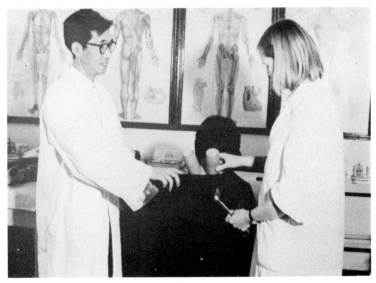

Cupping with Bamboo Cups.

Cupping is simply the use of partially evacuated glass or bamboo cups over the acupuncture point. A partial vacuum is created inside the cup by a flame, and with an adroit flick of the hand the cup is put on to the skin.

V. LENGTH OF TREATMENT

A course of treatment usually comprises eight sessions; these sessions are every day, or sometimes more frequently in acute diseases, but they may be less frequent in chronic diseases. More than one course of treatment may be needed and there should be a rest of a week or so between each course.

In the sections on each disease recommendations have been made when the rule of daily treatment does not apply.

In general two or three treatments are given to consolidate the effects of acupuncture (after the symptoms have gone), so strict adherence to the length of treatment may not be needed. In the West treatment is less frequent.

SECTION 3

THE THERAPY OF
SOME COMMON DISEASES

A. MUSCULO-SKELETAL DISEASES

ARTHRITIS

All types of arthritis are diseases of bi. Bi means a blocked or obstructed channel. This may be due to the invasion of a channel by a pathogen or due to direct damage to a channel, such as in a strain. When a channel is damaged there is poor circulation of qi and blood, and this will cause pain.

If the pain wanders then this is called *Wandering Bi* and it is due to invasion by wind. If it is painful then it is due to cold and is called *Painful Bi.* If there is a heavy feeling in the limbs and body, or in the part that is affected by the arthritis, then it is called *Heavy Bi* and it is due to invasion by damp. If a joint is hot then it is *Hot Bi* and it is due to the accumulation of wind, cold and damp, with the subsequent invasion of heat.

These types of bi are not mutually exclusive; there may be a heavy, painful bi or a wandering, hot bi.

Painful Heavy Bi
This is often seen in chronic arthritis, either rheumatoid or osteo-arthritis. There is slight swelling around the joints and the joints are sore, and the soreness will often become more intense on wet or cloudy days. There may be chronic malaise and a numb feeling in the affected joints and surrounding muscles. The tongue coating is thin, white and greasy, and the pulse is soft, thready and slow. This is due to invasion by cold and damp.

Wandering Hot Bi
This is often seen in acute rheumatoid or in acute rheumatic arthritis. If a single joint is hot and the bi does not wander then it may be a septic arthritis. The patient complains of fever and painful, red, swollen joints. There also may be limited joint movement, stiffness, a general lack of mobility, excessive sweating and irritability. The tongue coating is yellow and greasy and the pulse rapid. This is due to obstruction of the channels by wind and heat.

Painful Bi
This is seen in monoarthritis or local joint trauma, caused by the disruption of the channels. The pathogen that invades is usually cold, but this invasion is often only superficial and it may not produce any changes of the pulse or tongue.

Treatment

In heavy painful bi disperse the wind and cold and remove the obstruction, using the reinforcing method. Moxa or cupping should be used to disperse cold.

In wandering hot bi dispel the wind and resolve the damp and heat, thereby removing the obstruction in the channels. Use the reducing method.

In painful bi dispel the cold and remove the obstruction to the flow of qi. Use the reinforcing method. Moxa or cupping may also be useful.

Prescription

Initially use general points to correct the invasion by the pathogen and then use local points for the pain.

Cold Bi

Hegu LI 4   Zusanli St 36   Xuehai Sp 10
Qihai Ren 6

Hot Bi

Dazhui Du 14   Sanyinjiao Sp 6   Quchi LI 11
Zhigou SJ 6   Yinlingquan Sp 9   Xuanzhong GB 39

Painful Bi

Use local and distal points, as outlined in other sections, for each painful joint.

Points According to Symptoms

For *shoulder joint pain* use Jianyu (LI 15), Jugu (LI 16) and Jianliao (SJ 14).

For *elbow pain* use Quchi (LI 11), Shousanli (LI 10) and Shaohai (H 3).

For *wrist joint pain* use Waiguan (SJ 5), Yangchi (SJ 4) and Yangxi (LI 5).

For *pain in the phalangeal joints of hand* use Zhongzhu (SJ 3), Hegu (LI 4) and Baxie (Extra).

For *hip joint pain* use Femur-Juliao (GB 29) and Biguan (St 31).

For *knee joint pain* use Xiyan (Extra) and Lianqiu (St 34).

For *ankle joint pain* use Jiexi (St 41), Qiuxu (GB 40) and Kunlun (UB 60).

For *pain in the phalangeal joints of the foot* use Xingjian (Liv 2), Foot-Linqi (GB 41) and Bafeng (Extra).

For *pain in the lumbo dorsal region* use Jizhong (Du 6), Kunlun (UB 60), Weizhong (UB 40), Shenzhu (Du 12) and Mingmen (Du 4).

When there is *pain in the neck* use Houxi (SI 3) and Louzhen (Extra).

When there is *cold bi in the body* use Zhigou (SJ 6) and Xuanzhong (GB 39).

When there is *hot bi in the body* use Xiangu (St 43).

The Reasons for Point Selection

Hegu dispels wind and cold.

Xuehai tonifies blood and disperses cold (pi-spleen commands blood).

Zusanli and Qihai tonify and strengthen the body.

Dazhui and Quchi clear wind and heat.

Yinlingquan and Sanyinjiao resolve damp and clear heat.

Zhigou removes heat in the Sanjiao.

Xuanzhong is the influential point for the marrow.

Jizhong, Shenzhu and Mingmen command the yang qi of the body.

In any arthritic pain, or pain from any pathology, the pain may radiate from the site of damage. If the site of origin of the pain is not painful then it is only necessary to treat the radiation of the pain.

ACUTE AND CHRONIC BACK PAIN

Acute Sprain
This is often caused by sudden movement or by a strain while lifting a heavy weight. There is usually a pricking, fixed painful area in the lumbar region combined with severe limitation of back movements. This is caused by a direct injury to the channels of the back resulting in retardation of qi and stagnation of blood in those channels. The pulse and tongue are usually normal.

Cold and Damp
This presents as a dragging pain in the lower back, radiating to the hips or lower limbs. It is worse on cold, rainy, or cloudy days. The channels are blocked by damp, wind and cold, which may be caused by lying or sitting on damp, cold ground. The tongue proper is pale and the tongue coating is white and greasy, the pulse is xu.

Xu of Shen-kidney
This occurs when the patient is run down. There is a lingering ache in the lumbar region with weakness in the legs and knees. The pain is worse after activity and better after rest. Local pressure relieves the pain and cold worsens it. This is due to a deficiency of qi of shen-kidney. The tongue proper is pale and the tongue coating is deficient, the pulse is xu.

Treatment
In acute strain promote the circulation of qi and blood, remove the blood stasis and relieve pain.

In cold and damp, warm and remove the obstruction from the channels.

In xu of shen-kidney, tonify and reinforce the shen-kidney qi.

Prescription

Acute Sprain
Renzhong Du 26   Yaotongdian (Extra)

These two points may be used to relieve acute muscle spasm.

Occasionally pressure rather than needles may work on these points. The needles should be inserted into the points and manipulated strongly while the patient moves his back; this may be a painful process. If the pain is central use Renzhong, if it is on one side use Yaotongdian on the side of the pain. Local and distal points should then be used to consolidate treatment.

Cold and Damp
Shiqizhui (Extra)   Dachangshu UB 25   Shenshu UB 23
Yaoyangguan Du 3   Weizhong UB 40   Guanyuanshu UB 26

Ah shi points (these are useful and important in all chronic back pain).

Xu of Shen-kidney
Shenshu UB 23   Taixi K 3   Zhishi UB 52
Weizhong UB 40   Ah shi points

The general principles that govern chronic back pain are:
1. Look for internal organ dysfunction and treat if it is present.
2. Use local painful points, whether they are acupuncture points or Ah shi points, together with distal points, initially Weizhong and, if this is not effective, Kunlun.

Auricular Therapy
Lumbo-sacral vertebrae, shenmen.

SCIATICA

Sciatica results when the channels and collaterals are invaded by wind, cold and damp. This is because there is an insufficiency of normal qi, caused by an obstruction in the channels, and resulting in poor circulation of qi and blood. The symptoms are pain and soreness along the urinary bladder channel, tenderness at points Chengfu (UB 36), Weizhong (UB 40) and Kunlun (UB 60), difficulty in walking and pain intensified by sneezing and bending. The pulse is gliding, bow-string and tight, the tongue coating is white and greasy.

Treatment
Dispel the wind and cold and resolve damp. Free and invigorate the flow of qi in the channels and collaterals. Use the reducing method.

Prescription

Zhibian UB 54   Xingjan (Extra) (Third point in
Huantiao GB 30   equal: Δ with UB 54 and GB 29)
Chengfu UB 36   Yinmen UB 37
Weizhong UB 40   Chengshan UB 57
Kunlun UB 60

Points According to Symptoms
For *pain along lateral side of limb* add Fengshi (GB 31), Yanglingquan (GB 34) and Xuanzhong (GB 39).

For *pain in lumbar region* add Shenshu (UB 23) and Dachangshu (UB 25).

Huantiao (GB 30) is the most important point for sciatica, and it should always be used in every prescription.

Auricular Therapy
Sciatic nerve, buttocks, subcortex, shenmen.

Hand Acupuncture
Sciatica.

ARTHRITIS OF THE SHOULDER JOINT

A deficiency of normal qi and a weakness in defensive qi leads to invasion of wind, cold and damp in the channels over the shoulder. This causes retardation of qi and impairs its circulation, resulting in pain. Strain or trauma of the shoulder muscles can also lead to the same condition. The disease usually develops slowly and, as cold accumulates in the joint, adhesions are formed and a frozen or 'congealed' joint results. This develops in roughly three stages, early, middle and late.

Early Stage

This presents with unilateral soreness and limitation of movement. The soreness may radiate to the neck or into the deltoid muscle but there will be no obvious swelling or redness in the shoulder. Initially there is a mild limitation of movement, but this may progress if there is a further injury. This is due to the invasion of the channels by wind and damp, causing disharmony of qi.

Middle Stage

This presents with severe pain which is worse at night and often causes disturbed sleep. There is obvious swelling and distension in the deltoid muscle and there are tender spots near, or on, Jianneiling (Extra), Jianyu (LI 15), Tianzong (SI 11) and Binao (LI 14), and possibly other local points. This is due to the cold causing contraction of the muscles and obstruction to the flow of qi and blood.

Late Stage

This presents with severe limitation of shoulder movement and hard knobbly muscles in the shoulder area, with tender spots in the scapular and deltoid region. In very severe cases deltoid atrophy and a false acromion may appear and this is due to adhesions of the tendons and muscles around the joint.

There are two main types of late stage shoulder arthritis:

1. *Xu type.* This may accompany a chronic disease of the fei-lung or stomach and the patient will present with muscle atrophy locally. There will also be a weak constitution due to a chronic insufficiency of nourishing qi and blood and this makes the muscles and tendons deficient and atrophic.

2. *Shi type.* This is due to some sort of musculo-skeletal injury that causes invasion of cold and subsequent stagnation of qi and blood, leading to the formation of adhesions. This is a bi disease, there is no zang fu disease.

Treatment

Assess if the zang fu is abnormal and, if it is, treat it.

In the early stage: Dispel cold and disperse damp, therefore freeing the channels.

In the middle stage: Dispel wind and disperse damp, freeing the channels.

In the late stage: For the xu type, nourish the qi, free the tendons and ligaments and regulate the function of the channels. For the shi type, dispel cold, remove stagnation and free the channels.

Prescription

The common points for all shoulder pain are:

Jianyu LI 15   Jianliao SJ 14   Quchi LI 11

Binao LI 14   Jianneiling (Extra) (This point is 1 cun above the

Jugu LI 16   anterior axillary fold, midway between the fold
                    and Jianyu LI 15

Early Stage

Jianyu LI 15   Jianliao SJ 14   Quchi LI 11

Jianneiling (Extra)

Moxa may be used on the needles (warm needling), and the needles should be stimulated with the reducing method.

Middle Stage

Quyuan SI 13   Naoshu SI 10   Binao LI 14

Ah shi points. Moxa may be used on these points.

Auricular Therapy

Shoulder joint, shoulder, shenmen, adrenal.

Late Stage

For xu type treat the underlying organ pathology as well as the local points.

Jianneiling (Extra)   Jianyu LI 15   Dazhui Du 14

Jianjing GB 21   Ah shi points on scapular

Use Sanjian (LI 3) *for difficulty in raising the arm.*

Use Zhongzhu (SJ 3) *for difficult adduction.*

Use Houxi (SI 3) *for difficult abduction.*

Use Taiyuan (Lu 9) *for difficult internal rotation.*

It is important to use distal points with the local points in all three stages. Use Hegu (LI 4), Houxi (SI 3) or Waiguan (SJ 5), depending on which channel crosses the pain.

For an acute strain of the shoulder use Tiaokou (St 38) towards Chengshan (UB 57) while the patient moves the shoulder; this will remove acute muscle spasm.

ACUTE AND CHRONIC PAIN OF THE JOINTS ON THE FOUR EXTREMITIES

This is due to retardation of qi and stagnation of blood causing a disruption of the flow of qi in the channels and collaterals. This may be an acute strain or a chronic painful bi; they are dealt with together as the points used are the same.

Symptoms
There may be a soft tissue sprain around the ankle, knee, wrist or elbow, and this will present with a painful swollen joint that has limited or painful movement. If the pain is more chronic, due to osteoarthritis, the symptoms are often similar to acute strains. There will be localized tenderness, joint movement may be limited and there may also be joint swelling, or even a disordered joint. In both cases there may be marked tender spots; these should be treated whether they are acupuncture points or just Ah shi points.

Treatment
Assess if the zang fu is abnormal and, if it is, treat it. Promote the circulation of blood and qi by removing the obstruction.

Prescription

Wrist Joint
Yangxi LI 5	Yangchi SJ 4	Shenmen H 7
Taiyuan Lu 9	Yanggu SI 5	

Elbow Joint
Quchi LI 11	Quze P 3	Tianjing SJ 10
Shousanli LI 10	Xiaohai SI 8	Shaohai H 3
Waiguan SJ 5		

Ankle Joint

Jiexi St 41	Qiuxu GB 40	Kunlun UB 60
Taixi K 3	Shangqui Sp 5	Zhaohai K 6

Knee Joint

Xiyan (Extra)		Yinlingquan Sp 9	Weizhong UB 40
Zusanli St 36		

See also osteoarthritis of the knee.

If the strain is an acute one then a channel balancing method may be applied. This means that the area on the unaffected limb, equivalent to the painful area, can be treated. If there is acute pain use strong stimulation of the needle.

Auricular Therapy

This is most effective for acute pain. Use the area on the ear that represents the painful area on the body, i.e. wrist, elbow, knee or ankle, and exercise the affected area while stimulating the needle.

TENOSYNOVITIS

This is due to the channels and collaterals being invaded by wind and cold, causing stagnation and retardation of qi. Local pain is the main symptom.

Treatment

Assess if there is any zang fu disorder and treat it if one is present. Promote the circulation of blood and qi by removing the stagnation of blood, freeing the channels and collaterals.

1. *Flexor digitorum tenosynovitis*

Prescription

Select painful spots as the main points matched with:

Lieque Lu 7	Yangxi LI 5	Ah shi point

Use Moxa on the Ah shi point.

2. *Tennis elbow*

Prescription
Select painful spot as the main point.

Quchi LI 11 Waiguan SJ 5
Ah shi point (Or distal point of another channel if the
 Ah shi point is on another channel.)

Use moxa on the Ah shi point.

STRAINED NECK

This is an injury of the jin. It is due to obstruction of the channels by wind and cold, causing poor circulation of qi and blood.

Symptoms
The patient presents with an acute muscular pain in the neck, accompanied by limitation of neck movement. There is a dragging pain in the shoulders and neck and there may be a headache or a chill. The tongue coating is thin and white and the pulse is tight.

Treatment
Assess if there is any zang fu disorder and, if there is, treat it. Remove the obstruction, dispel wind and disperse cold; use the reducing method.

Prescription
Fengchi GB 20 Tianzhu UB 10
Houxi SI 3 Waiguan SJ 5
Ah Shi points Hegu LI 4

Hand Acupuncture
Use Luozhen (Extra) and Zhongzhu (SJ 3). Manipulate the needles while the patient moves his neck.

Auricular Therapy
Shenmen, neck, cervical vertebrae.

HIP PAIN

This is most frequently due to osteoarthritis of the hip. If there is internal organ disease then treat it along with local and distal points for the hip, otherwise treat hip pain as a painful bi. In diseases of pain it is not always necessary to treat the pathology, but it is more important to treat the pain; this is often illustrated very clearly by hip pain. The pain may be generated from the hip, but it may present as knee pain. It is therefore necessary to treat the site of actual pain using local points around the knee, even though the pain may be coming from a damaged hip.

Prescription
Biguan St 31   Femur-Juliao GB 29 Huantiao GB 30
Fengshi GB 31   Zhibian UB 54
Ah shi points.

Use distal points on the channel over which the pain radiates.

For *pain down the stomach channel* use Neiting St 44.

For *pain down the urinary bladder channel* use Weizhong UB 40 or Kunlun UB 60.

For *pain down the gall bladder channel* use Yanglingquan GB 34.

Insert the needles deeply.

Auricular Therapy
Hip, Shenmen.

KNEE PAIN

This is a disease of bi and the signs of each type of bi are discussed in the section on arthritis. This pain is often due to osteoarthritis of the knee, but acute strains will respond to the same points.

Treatment
Assess if there is any zang fu disease and, if there is, treat it. Resolve the pathogen causing the bi and remove the obstruction to the channels.

Prescription
Important points that are often used are:

Xiyan (Extra)	Yinlingquan Sp 9	Weizhong UB 40

Other points may be used, dependent on the area of tenderness:

Heding (Extra)	Zusanli St 36	Dubi St 35
Lianqiu St 34	Yanglingquan GB 34	
Ah shi points		

Change the points if any become painful and use moxa on the needle if the damage is chronic and due to the congealing action of cold.

Auricular Therapy
Knee, Shenmen.

CERVICAL SPONDYLOSIS

This is a disease of bi and each type of bi is discussed in the section on arthritis.

Treatment
Assess if there is any zang fu disease and treat it. Resolve the pathogen causing the bi and remove the obstruction to the flow of qi and blood in the channels.

Prescription
Commonly used points are:

Fengchi GB 20	Jianjing GB 21	Dazhui Du 14
Quchi LI 11	Waiguan SJ 5	Ah shi points

Other points may also be used dependent on the radiation of the pain, they are:

Huatuojiaji (Extra)	Dashu UB 11	Kunlun UB 60
Yamen Du 15	Houxi SI 3	Tianzong SI 11
Quyuan SI 13	Jianwaishu SI 14	

Auricular Therapy
Cervical vertebrae, neck, Shenmen.

B. DISEASES OF THE NERVOUS SYSTEM

SEQUELAE OF CEREBROVASCULAR ACCIDENTS

Excess of the Yang of Gan-liver
This is caused by the shen-kidney (water) failing to nourish the gan-liver (wood), leading to an excess of the yang of gan-liver. It may also be caused by an excess of anger leading to an excess of the yang of the liver. A lack of rest may also cause insufficiency of yin, again resulting in an excess of yang. This kind of stroke is usually of abrupt onset and affects the mind, the pulse is bowstring and the tongue proper is red, with a deficient coating. It is caused by an excess of yang (wind) resulting in the ascent of qi and blood, which congeals and stagnates in the head.

Excess of Phlegm and Damp
Obesity, eating fatty foods, and irregular feeding, all lead to the invasion of damp and the production of phlegm. An excess of phlegm and damp turn into heat, and heat leads to wind. The wind causes an ascent of blood and qi and this congeals and stagnates in the head, causing obstruction of the channels. This type of stroke is usually of slow onset, the patient is often obese and likes fatty foods. It is a less severe stroke than an excess of the yang of gan-liver and the mind is not usually affected. The tongue coating is thick and greasy and the pulse is bowstring and sometimes thready.

Shi Type
This is often a combination of the above two in the acute stage, one type being usually predominant. There is a short duration of illness, dizziness, vertigo, limb paralysis, excess sputum and difficulty in speaking. The tongue coating is thin, yellow and greasy, the pulse is bowstring and gliding, or bowstring and thready.

Xu Type
This is the chronic result of a stroke and it develops after some weeks. It is usually a combination of the above types. There is a flaccid hemiplegia, dyspnoea, lassitude, muscle wasting and, chronically, there may be spasm and spasticity of the muscles. The tongue coating is thin and white, the tongue proper is light coloured and the pulse is thready. This is due to an insufficiency of qi and blood and obstruction of the channels.

Treatment

In excess of yang, pacify the gan-liver and remove the obstruction in the channels.

In phlegm and damp, resolve the phlegm and damp and remove the obstruction in the channels.

In shi type a combination of the above treatments is needed.

In xu type, reinforce and tonify the qi and blood and remove the obstruction in the channels.

Prescription

Excess of Yang

Hegu LI 4	Taixi K 3	Taichong Liv 3
Ganshu UB 18	Yanglingquan GB 34	

Excess of Phlegm and Damp

Hegu LI 4	Pishu UB 20	Fenglong St 40
Sanyinjiao Sp 6	Waiguan SJ 5	

Shi Type

Combination of above.

Xu Type

Shenshu UB 23	Jianyu LI 15	Quchi LI 11
Shousanli LI 10	Waiguan SJ 5	Hegu LI 4
Huantiao GB 30	Fengshi GB 31	Zusanli St 36
Yanglingquan GB 34	Xuanzhong GB 39	Jiexi St 41

Points According to Symptoms

For *facial palsy* see the treatment for facial paralysis.

For *aphasia and a stiff tongue* use Lianquan (Ren 23), Zhaohai (K 6) and Tongli (H 5).

For *arm spasticity* use Chize (Lu 5), Neiguan (P 6), and Shaohai (H 3).

For *leg spasticity* use Sanyinjiao (Sp 6), Taixi (K 3), and Jiexi (St 41).

For *shoulder and hip pain* use Jianneiling (Extra), Jianliao (SJ 14) (shoulder), Biguan (St 31), and Femur-juliao (GB 29) (hip).

To lower blood pressure use Quchi (LI 11), Hegu (LI 4) and Taichong (Liv 3). If the blood pressure is still high then use Taixi (K 3) alone.

The Reasons for Point Selection
Taichong pacifies the gan-liver and eliminates wind.

Ganshu and Yanglingquan eliminate the wind of the gan-liver.

Taixi regulates the shen-kidney.

Fenglong resolves sputum.

Waiguan regulates the middle jiao and removes damp.

Jianyu, Quchi, Hegu and Zusanli reinforce and tonify qi and blood and remove obstruction.

Local and distal points free the flow of qi in the affected channels.

Treat daily for three months on the affected side, then every other day. If there is not a complete reversal of symptoms after six months then treat on the unaffected side.

Scalp Acupuncture
Scalp acupuncture is probably better than body acupuncture for strokes and many other causes of spasticity such as severe head injuries. It seems to increase the local blood supply to the damaged part of the brain so do not use it until at least two weeks after a stroke. Put needles into the areas that represent function impairment in the patient, and stimulate these areas electrically.

Use the motor region for motor impairment and motor aphasia.

Use the sensory region for sensory impairment.

Use the foot motor sensory region for functional impairment of the lower limb.

Use the speech region 2 for sensory aphasia.

Use the speech region 3 for nominal aphasia.

Use the vertigo region for hearing and balance problems.

Treat regularly for about ten sessions in each course, and give as many courses of treatment as the patient needs. When there is no further improvement stop treatment.

HEADACHE

Headaches may be due to exogenous factors such as wind and heat, or wind and cold. They can also be caused by endogenous factors such as hyperactivity of yang of the gan-liver.

Excess anger depresses the qi of the gan-liver and causes an ascent of fire, giving rise to headaches. There may also be xu, or deficiency of blood. This causes headaches because the brain has an inadequate circulation of qi and blood. When phlegm and damp invade the pi-spleen this is usually due to obesity and over-eating, and the pathogens that invade may ascend to affect the head and cause headaches.

Exogenous Factors
This often occurs after a common cold, there is a dislike of cold or heat, and a cough. The tongue coating is thin and white, and the pulse is rapid and floating.

Endogenous Factors
Hyperactivity of Yang
This presents with dizziness, irritability, a flushed face and a pounding headache. Visual disturbances often occur prior to the headache and there is usually some photophobia during the headache. The tongue coating is thin and yellow and the pulse is bowstring. In Western medicine this is called migraine.

Xu of Blood
This presents with lassitude, palpitations, pallor, and a dull continuous headache. The tongue coating is thin and white, the tongue proper white, and the pulse is thready soft and forceless.

Phlegm and Damp
This presents with a feeling of fullness and distension in the chest, abdomen and head, associated with nausea and vomiting. The tongue coating is white and greasy and the pulse is gliding.

Treatment
If exogenous factors are present then dispel the wind and disperse the cold and heat. In the endogenous causes of headache, pacify the gan-liver in hyperactivity of yang, tonify qi and blood in xu of

blood, and strengthen the pi-spleen and resolve damp when the headaches are due to the invasion of phlegm and damp.

Prescription

Exogenous Factors
Dazhui Du 14   Quchi LI 11   Hegu LI 4
Waiguan SJ 5

Endogenous Factors

Hyperactivity of Yang of Gan-liver
Taichong Liv 3   Ququan Liv 8   Yanglingquan GB 34

Xu of Blood
Qihai Ren 6   Zusanli St 36

Phlegm and Damp
Fenglong St 40   Sanyinjiao Sp 6

Points According to Symptoms
For a *frontal headache* use Yangbai (GB 14), and Yintang (Extra).

For a *migraine* use the tender points on the gall bladder channel, Taiyang (Extra), Touwei (St 8), and Shuaigu (GB 8).

For *occipital headaches* use Fengchi (GB 20), and Kunlun (UB 60).

For *vertical headaches* use Baihui (Du 20) and Neiguan (P 6).

The Reasons for Point Selection
Dazhui, Quchi, Hegu and Waiguan disperse wind, cold and heat.

Taichong, Yanglingquan and Ququan pacify the gan-liver.

Qihai and Zusanli strengthen the body and tonify the qi and blood.

Fenglong and Sanyinjiao strengthen the pi-spleen and stomach, and resolve damp.

The points used for symptoms also help to promote the circulation of qi and blood and therefore resolve the obstruction.

Auricular Therapy
Forehead, Occiput, Taiyang, Brain stem, Shenmen, Sub-cortex.

If a headache is due to a brain tumour then acupuncture usually makes it much worse.

FACIAL NERVE PARALYSIS

This is due to the invasion of the channels and collaterals by wind and cold, causing an obstruction of qi and blood. The signs are deviation of the mouth and eyes, ptosis, saliva dribbling from the corner of the mouth, and impaired facial movement on the affected side. There may also be pain behind the root of the ear. The tongue coating is thin and white, and the pulse floating and tight.

Treatment
Dispel the cold and wind and remove the obstruction from the channels and collaterals. Use the reducing method. If the patient has muscle spasm use the reinforcing method. When the patient has a headache and pain behind the ear facial paralysis is more difficult to treat. Use Yifeng (SJ 17) to alleviate the pain and the facial paralysis will become easier to treat.

Prescription
Select points from the Yangming (large intestine and stomach) channels as qi and blood are abundant in these channels.

Yifeng SJ 17	Quanliao SI 18	Yangbai GB 14
Taiyang (Extra)	Dicang St 4	Jiache St 6
Hegu LI 4	Taichong Liv 3	

Points According to Symptoms
For *headache* add Fengchi (GB 20).

For *a slanting upper labial groove* add Renzhong (Du 26).

The Reasons for Point Selection
Yifeng has a strong action in removing obstructions and dispelling wind. Use deep puncture.

Yangbai, Taiyang, and Quanliao are all situated on facial nerves and they free and invigorate qi and blood in the local areas.

Jiache and Dicang dispel wind and remove obstruction.

Taichong and Hegu are distal points and they both disperse wind.

For patients with chronic facial paralysis use cupping on Quanliao (SI 18).

Use points on the affected side, except for Hegu (LI 4) and Taichong (Liv 3), which should be used bilaterally.

If there is no result after one course of treatment use moxa on ginger and then, if necessary, use electro-acupuncture.

TRIGEMINAL NEURALGIA

This is due to either invasion of wind and cold causing an obstruction of the channels and collaterals, or flaring up of fire of both the gan-liver and stomach. The gan-liver is over-active because of a deficiency of yin and a hyperactivity of yang.

Invasion of Wind and Cold
This causes a paroxysmal pricking or burning pain on the face, and a dislike of cold. The tongue coating is thin and white and the pulse is floating, or floating and rapid.

Fire of Xu Nature
This causes an intermittent burning sensation on the face and irritability. The tongue coating is thin and yellow, and the pulse is bowstring and rapid.

Treatment
When there is invasion of wind and cold, dispel the wind and cold and invigorate and free the qi and blood in the channels. When there is a fire of xu nature, sedate the yang of the gan-liver and stomach.

Prescription
Invasion of wind and cold:
Hegu LI 4   Waiguan SJ 5

Fire of xu nature:
Neiting St 44   Taichong Liv 3

Points According to Symptoms
For *pain in the first branch* (opthalmic branch) of the fifth nerve use Taiyang (Extra), Yangbai (GB 14) and Zanzhu (UB 2).

For *pain in the second branch* (maxillary branch) of the fifth nerve use Sibai (St 2), Quanliao (SI 18) and Yingxiang (LI 20).

For *pain in the third branch* (mandibular branch) of the fifth nerve use Xianguan (St 7), Jiache (St 6) and Dicang (St 4).

The Reasons for Point Selection
Hegu and Waiguan dispel wind and cold.

Neiting and Taichong disperse the fire of the stomach and gan-liver.

NEURASTHENIA

Neurasthenia is a symptom complex that includes much of what we think of as anxiety and depression. It may affect the organs of the pi-spleen, xin-heart, gan-liver and shen-kidney. Overjoy, fear or fright affects the xin-heart, excessive anger affects the gan-liver and exceqsive anxiety, grief or on-kidney. Overjoy, fear or fright affects the xin-heart, excessive anger affects the gan-liver and excessive anxiety, grief or overthinking (including overwork) will affect the pi-spleen. A long chronic illness will affect the pi-spleen, the shen-kidney and the xin-heart.

Xu Type
This is rather like a depression. It presents with insomnia, sleep disturbance, vertigo, poor memory, palpitations, anorexia, lassitude, lumbar ache, tinnitus and blurred vision. The tongue coating is thin and white, the tongue proper is pale, the pulse is soft, thready and forceless.

This is due to xu of xin-heart, and pi-spleen because there is a xu of shen-kidney.

Shi Type
This is more like an anxiety state. It presents with dizziness,

vertigo, headache and a feeling of distension in the head, insomnia, irritability, pain and distension in the costal and hypochondriac region, and tinnitus. The tongue coating is thin and white, the tongue proper is red and the pulse is thready and bowstring. This is due to depression of the qi of the gan-liver leading to hyperactivity of the yang of gan-liver, and an excess of fire that affects the mind.

Treatment
In the xu type tonify the xin-heart and pi-spleen, and nourish the yin of the shen-kidney.

In the shi type invigorate and relieve the depression of qi and pacify the gan-liver.

Prescription
Xu Type

Neiguan P 6	Shenmen H 7	Zusanli St 36
Yintang (Extra)	Sanyinjiao Sp 6	Taixi K 3
Fuliu K 7		

Shi Type

Hegu LI 4	Zhigou SJ 6	Sanyinjiao Sp 6
Yinglingquan Sp 9	Taichong Liv 3	Fengchi GB 20
Zhongfeng Liv 4		

Points According to Symptoms
For *discomfort in the epigastrium* use Zhongwan (Ren 12).

For *impotence* use Guanyuan (Ren 4) and Zhongji (Ren 3).

The Reasons for Point Selection
Neiguan, Shenmen and Yintang calm the mind and soothe the mentality.

Zusanli and Sanyinjiao tonify the pi-spleen and stomach.

Taixi and Fuliu nourish the yin of the shen-kidney.

Zhigou and Hegu invigorate qi and resolve depression.

Taichong and Zhongfeng pacify the gan-liver.

INNER AURAL VERTIGO

Vertigo is caused by obstruction of the middle jiao with phlegm and damp. This occurs when qi is deficient and the pi-spleen fails to take charge of transportation and transformation. Phlegm and damp then obstruct the middle jiao and rise to disturb the clear palace of the mind. When the qi of the shen-kidney is deficient there is a weakness of the lower extremities, and this is associated with vertigo.

Obstruction of the Middle Jiao by Phlegm and Damp
This presents with dizziness, vertigo, blurred vision, anorexia, distension in the abdomen and chest, and lassitude. The tongue coating is white and greasy and the pulse is soft.

Xu of Shen-kidney
This presents with dizziness, vertigo, blurred vision, a lumbar ache, weakness of the legs and a pale face. The tongue proper is pale, the tongue coating is deficient and the pulse is thready.

Treatment
Obstruction of the middle jiao should be treated by strengthening the pi-spleen, resolving damp and tonifying the qi. Use the reducing method. Xu of shen-kidney should be treated by tonifying the shen-kidney and the qi. Use the reinforcing method with moxa.

Prescription

Obstruction of Middle Jiao by Phlegm and Damp
Fengchi GB 20	Neiguan P 6	Sanyinjiao Sp 6
Pishu UB 20	Zhongwan Ren 12	Fenglong St 40

Xu of Shen-kidney
Shenshu UB 23	Taixi K 3	Fuliu K 7
Shenmen H 7	Fengchi GB 20	Zhongwan Ren 12
Guanyuan Ren 4		

Points According to Symptoms
For *tinnitus* add Yifeng (SJ 17) and Tinghui (GB 2).

For *spermatorrhea* add Zhishi (UB 52).

The Reasons for Point Selection
Shenmen, Fengchi, Neiguan and Sanyinjiao act as sedative points. They also stop vomiting and relieve vertigo.

Pishu and Zhongwan strengthen the pi-spleen, regulate the stomach and stop adverse ascending of qi.

Taixi, Fuliu and Shenshu tonify the shen-kidney and the original qi.

Guanyuan strengthens the body's resistance against disease.

ENURESIS

Enuresis is due to xu of shen-kidney and pi-spleen. Insufficiency of the qi of shen-kidney results in a lack of control of urine. Insufficiency of the qi of pi-spleen causes the qi to fall, also causing a lack of control of urine.

Treatment
Reinforce the yang of shen-kidney and tonify the pi-spleen. Use the reinforcing method.

Prescription
Guanyuan Ren 4	Qihai Ren 6	Sanyinjiao Sp 6
Taixi K 3		

or back points:
Shenshu UB 23	Pishu UB 20
Zhishi UB 52	Baihui Du 20

The Reasons for Point Selection
Shenshu, Pishu, Taixi, Zhishi and Sanyinjiao all reinforce the shen-kidney, tonify the qi and strengthen the function of pi-spleen.

Qihai and Guanyuan strengthen the body's resistance and help the function of the urinary bladder in controlling the urine.

Auricular Therapy
Urinary bladder, Shenmen.

Hand Acupuncture
Nocturia, 1 and 2.

C. GENERAL MEDICINE

GASTRIC AND DUODENAL ULCERS

This presents with pain in the epigastric region and it is due to dysfunction of the pi-spleen, the gan-liver or the stomach, or a combination of these organs.

Pi-spleen
In obese patients, or people with a weak asthenic constitution, cold invades very easily and this causes the accumulation of food and drink in the stomach and small intestine. This process affects the function of transportation and transformation, and causes a decline of yang in the middle jiao. Ultimately this may result in haematemesis, or perforation of the ulcer.

Gan-liver
Depression or anger may impair the freeing function of the gan-liver and the qi of the gan-liver may then invade the stomach.

Stomach
Irregular feeding, or too much cold or uncooked food, leads to a malfunction of the stomach and nvasion by various pathogens.

Xu Type
This presents with vague epigastric pain relieved by food or hot drinks, there may be heartburn and cold extremities. The pain can be relieved by pressure. The tongue coating is thin and white and the pulse is thready, weak and forceless. This is due to xu of pi-spleen allowing invasion of cold, causing a disturbance of the yang in the middle jiao and resulting in a peptic ulcer.

Shi Type
This presents with a full, bursting epigastric pain. The pain is worse when it is pressed and there may be associated irritability, flatulence, restlessness and heartburn, as well as a reduced food intake. The tongue coating is thin and white and the pulse is bowstring. This is due to depression of the gan-liver and retardation of qi, which allows the qi of the gan-liver to invade the stomach and cause an ulcer.

Treatment

In the xu type strengthen the pi-spleen and regulate the function of the stomach, warm the middle jiao and disperse the cold. Reinforcing method and cupping, plus moxa, should be used.

In the shi type promote the freeing function of the gan-liver and strength its qi, regulate the stomach and stop adverse ascending of qi. Use the reducing method.

Prescription

Xu Type

Zhongwan Ren 12	Neiguan P 6	Jianli Ren 11
Zusanli St 36	Sanyinjiao Sp 6	

Or back points:

Pishu UB 20	Weishu UB 21

Shi Type

Qimen Liv 14	Taichong Liv 3	Gongsun Sp 4
Yanglingquan GB 34	Liangmen St 21	

Or back points:

Pishu UB 20	Ganshu UB 18

Points According to Symptoms

For *nausea* use Neiguan (P 6).

For *severe gastric pain* use Liangqiu (St 34).

Between attacks put moxa on Zusanli (St 36); this will reduce the frequency of attacks.

The Reasons for Point Selection

Neiguan and Zusanli work together to stop pain and nausea.

Pishu and Weishu strengthen and regulate the pi-spleen.

Zhongwan is the influential point of the fu organs, it warms and strengthens the middle jiao.

Jianli strengthens the pi-spleen.

Sanyinjiao strengthens the pi-spleen.

Ganshu, Qimen and Taichong all promote the freeing function of the gan-liver.

Gongsun regulates the stomach and stops the adverse ascending of qi.

Liangqiu has a marked affect on acute pain.

ACUTE GASTROENTERITIS

This is usually seen in the summer and autumn. It presents with vomiting, diarrhoea, colicky abdominal pain, pallor, sweats and headache. When there is severe dehydration there may be numb, cold limbs. The tongue coating is white and thin or yellow, the pulse is rapid and gliding.

The stomach and pi-spleen are invaded by summer heat and damp, or they may be injured by the intake of contaminated food. This damages the transportation and transformation of food by the pi-spleen. Adverse ascent of qi causes vomiting, and descent of qi causes diarrhoea, if this activity becomes too violent then the body fluid is consumed and yang qi declines. This causes collapse and dehydration.

Treatment
Eliminate damp and heat and free the stagnation and retardation of qi. Use the reducing method.

Prescription
Neiguan P 6	Tianshu St 25	Zusanli St 36
Neiting St 44	Zhongwan Ren 12	Weizhong UB 40

The Reasons for Point Selection
Neiguan stops adverse ascent of qi (vomiting).

Zhongwan, Tianshu and Zusanli free and regulate the intestines.

Neiting and Weizhong dominate the body temperature and eliminate heat.

Acute gastroenteritis should be treated every four hours for about thirty minutes each treatment. Continue treating until the symptoms clear.

Hand Acupuncture
Gastroenteritis.

Auricular Therapy
Large intestine, lower portion of rectum, spleen.

CHRONIC ENTERITIS

This is related to pi-spleen and shen-kidney. Cold invades and causes a xu of pi-spleen which impairs the descent of qi and allows it to be lost in the stool. As there is a lack of nourishing qi the shen-kidney is injured and a lack of normal qi results.

This presents with chronic diarrhoea, lassitude, poor appetite, lumbar soreness and a cold sensation in the limbs. The tongue coating is thin and greasy and the pulse is soft and thready.

Treatment
Warm the middle jiao and strengthen the pi-spleen and shen-kidney. Use the reinforcing method and moxa.

Prescription
Qihai Ren 6	Zusanli St 36	Sanyinjiao Sp 6
Guanyuan Ren 4	Tianshu St 25	

Or back points:
Pishu UB 20	Shenshu UB 23

For an acute exacerbation add Shangjuxu (St 37).

The Reasons for Point Selection
Qihai, Guanyuan and Zusanli strengthen the body resistance against disease, tonify the pi-spleen and regulate the stomach.

Sanyinjiao tonifies the pi-spleen.

Tianshu is the front mu point for the large intestine and regulates the large intestine.

Pishu strengthens the pi-spleen.

Shenshu warms the shen-kidney.

Shangjuxu is a xi-cleft point, and these are always useful in acute diseases.

ACUTE DYSENTERY

This is caused by the invasion of summer heat and damp, or the intake of contaminated food. This may cause an acute infection or a chronic enteritis. The acute infection has a similar pathological mechanism to that of gastroenteritis, but it is more severe.

Damp and Heat
This presents with abdominal pain, pus and mucus in the stool, diarrhoea, abdominal distension, anorexia, irritability, a dry mouth, scanty dark yellow urine, and fever. The tongue coating is greasy and yellow and the pulse is gliding and rapid. This is caused by damp and heat invading the intestines and causing a malfunction of the transmission of normal qi by the pi-spleen. The qi of the fu organs is retarded and deficient.

Damp and Cold
This is the more chronic aftermath that can be left after the acute stage. It may also occur spontaneously. It presents with pus and blood in the stool, vague abdominal pain and clear profuse urine. The tongue coating is greasy and white and the pulse is soft and slow, or thready and slow.

This is due to invasion of the intestines and pi-spleen by damp and cold, causing a stagnation of the qi of the fu organs.

Treatment
In damp and heat expel the heat and eliminate the damp, regulating the flow of qi and blood. Use the reducing method.

In damp and cold warm the middle jiao and eliminate damp. This removes the stagnation of qi. Use the reducing method and moxa.

Prescription

Damp and Heat
Tianshu St 25   Shangjuxu St 37

Damp and Cold
Tianshu St 25   Zusanli St 36   Dachangshu UB 25

Points According to Symptoms

For *fever* add Dazhui (Du 14) and Quchi (LI 11).

For *nausea and vomiting* add Neiguan (P 6) and Zhongwan (Ren 12).

The Reasons for Point Selection

Tianshu is the front mu point for the large intestine and regulates the function of the large intestine.

Dachangshu and Shangjuxu promote the circulation of qi in the intestines.

Quchi and Dazhui remove heat.

Zusanli dissipates cold and frees the flow of qi.

Treat two to three times a day in the acute stages, then less as the disease is brought under control.

Auricular Therapy

Large intestine, lower portion of the rectum, spleen.

BILIARY TRACT DISEASE

The classical symptoms of biliary tract disease are hypochondriac pain and jaundice.

Stasis of the Liver and Gall Bladder

This presents with a bursting pain in the right hypochondrium and costal region, which radiates to the back and shoulders. There is often nausea, vomiting, flatulence and a stuffy feeling in the chest, and these feelings are intensified by emotional changes. The tongue coating is thin and white and the pulse is bowstring.

This is caused by the mental pathogen 'emotional upset', which alters the freeing function of the gan-liver causing stagnation of bile and impairment of the function of the pi-spleen. When bile is obstructed and qi is retarded stasis in the gan-liver and gall bladder results.

Accumulation of Damp and Heat
This is more like an acute cholecystitis. It presents with severe colicky pain in the right hypochondrium, fever, jaundice, yellow-red urine and dry hard stool. The tongue coating is yellow and greasy, the tongue proper is red and the pulse is bowstring and rapid.

This is caused by irregular feeding resulting in an impairment of pi-spleen. Damp then accumulates and turns into heat and this disturbs the freeing function of the gan-liver and gall bladder, resulting in the congealing of bile into stones. The subsequent retardation of qi, and stagnation of blood, cause the jaundice and fever.

Treatment
In stasis of the gan-liver free the gan-liver.

In accumulation of damp and heat remove the damp and eliminate the heat.

Prescription
The points used are basically the same for each type, but points are added for the symptoms of fever or nausea.

Yanglingquan GB 34   Zhigou SJ 6   Qimen Liv 14
Riyue GB 24   Dannang (Extra)   Burong St 19
Taichong Liv 3

Points According to Symptoms
For *vomiting* add Neiguan (P 6).

For *abdominal distension* add Zusanli (St 36).

For *fever* add Quchi (LI 11).

For *jaundice or shoulder-tip pain* add Ganshu (UB 18) and Danshu (UB 19).

The Reasons for Point Selection
Yanglingquan, Taichong, Qimen, Riyue and Zhigou all promote the freeing function of the gan-liver.

Neiguan and Zusanli regulate the stomach and stop vomiting.

Ganshu and Danshu free the gall bladder and eliminate jaundice.

Quchi eliminates heat and inflammation.

It is important to mention that the Chinese were using acupuncture to cause the discharge of quite large (one square centimetre) gall stones in the stool. This was achieved by using Qimen (Liv 14) and Riyue (GB 24) daily with electro-acupuncture, and then giving magnesium containing laxatives to clear the bowel. The stool was then sieved and the gall stones recovered.

The Chinese were beginning to collect some detailed figures on this method but our impression, and their initial results, seemed to show a tiny requirement for operative intervention in both acute and chronic biliary disease due to gall stones. This initial work did not have the depth and length of follow-up to draw any very dramatic conclusions, but it is of great interest.

ACUTE AND CHRONIC BRONCHITIS

Acute Bronchitis

Wind and Cold
This presents with chill, fever, a cough with watery sputum, and a general malaise. The tongue coating is thin, white and greasy and the pulse is floating. This is due to the invasion of the fei-lung by wind and cold, blocking the respiratory tract and impairing the normal ascent of qi of fei-lung. It is equivalent to a viral infection of the respiratory tract.

Wind and Heat
When invasion by heat occurs there is a high fever and a productive cough with yellow or green sputum. The tongue coating is yellow and thin, or yellow and greasy, and the pulse is rapid and floating. The fei-lung has been invaded by wind and heat, and phlegm and humour are then produced as secondary pathogens. This obstructs the absorption and descent of clean qi. It is equivalent to a bacterial chest infection.

Chronic Bronchitis
Acupuncture can only alleviate the symptoms of chronic bronchitis, it cannot cure the disease. Points should be used to

cause bronchodilation and also to tonify the shen-kidney and pi-spleen, or sedate the gan-liver, as these organs are often diseased.

Treatment
In wind and cold remove these pathogens and resolve the phlegm and obstruction in the fei-lung.

In wind and heat resolve the pathogens and remove the obstruction and phlegm.

In chronic bronchitis tonify the pi-spleen and shen-kidney, stop the cough and resolve the phlegm.

Prescription

Acute Bronchitis

Wind and Cold

Fengmen UB 12	Feishu UB 13	Lieque Lu 7
Chize Lu 5	Fenglong St 40	

Wind and Heat

Fengmen UB 12	Feishu UB 13	Dazhui Du 14
Taiyuan Lu 9	Quchi LI 11	Fenglong St 40

Chronic Bronchitis

Feishu UB 13	Fenglong St 40	Shenshu UB 23
Pishu UB 20	Taixi K 3	Taiyuan Lu 9
Sanyinjiao Sp 6	Taichong Liv 3	

In diseases of cold it is important to warm with moxa or cupping.

Points According to Symptoms
For an itchy throat use Tiantu (Ren 22).

For asthenia use Gaohuang (UB 43).

It is obviously not possible to use all these points at the same time, especially for chronic bronchitis. Feishu (UB 13) and Fenglong (St 40) should always be used and other points added as required. If there is an asthmatic element then consider the points discussed in that section.

The Reasons for Point Selection

Fengmen, Feishu, Lieque, Taiyuan and Chize free the qi of fei-lung and resolve phlegm.

Dazhui and Quchi resolve heat.

Fenglong and Sanyinjiao tonify the pi-spleen and eliminate phlegm.

Shenshu and Taixi tonify the shen-kidney.

Taichong sedates the gan-liver.

ASTHMA

Bronchial asthma is related to fei-lung, pi-spleen and shen-kidney. Invasion by the pathogens wind and heat, or wind and cold, causes stagnation of the qi of fei-lung. The qi cannot distribute the body fluid and the fluid then turns into phlegm. Irregular feeding or too much cold food causes a malfunction of pi-spleen and this leads to the production of phlegm.

In xu of shen-kidney there is an impairment of the intake of clean qi and this again causes a failure in distribution of the body fluid, and the subsequent production of phlegm.

Cold in Nature

This presents with a tight wheezy cough and white frothy sputum. The tongue coating is white and slippery and the pulse is floating and tight. This is due to the accumulation of phlegm and humour in the fei-lung blocking the respiratory tract and therefore blocking the normal ascent of qi.

Hot in Nature

This is an acute chest infection superimposed on asthma. There is a wheeze with thick yellow sputum, there may also be thirst and a fever. The tongue coating is yellow and greasy and the tongue proper is red, the pulse is gliding and rapid or bowstring and gliding. This is due to the accumulation of phlegm and invasion of heat into fei-lung impairing the function of dissipation and descent of clean qi.

Xu Nature

This is a more chronic syndrome, there is dyspnoea on slight exertion and a feeble cough, the face is yellow, there may be palpitations and central cyanosis. The tongue coating is thin, white and greasy, the tongue proper is light and the pulse is fine, soft and feeble. This is due to a deficiency of both shen-kidney and fei-lung, and the accumulation of phlegm.

Treatment

In cold asthma warm the fei-lung, dispel cold and resolve the phlegm.

In hot asthma remove the heat and resolve the phlegm.

In xu asthma tonify the fei-lung and shen-kidney and resolve the phlegm.

Prescription

Cold in Nature

Fengmen UB 12	Feishu UB 13	Tiantu Ren 22
Dingchuan (Extra)	Shanzhong Ren 17	Taiyuan Lu 9

Heat in Nature

Dingchuan (Extra)	Tiantu Ren 22	Fenglong St 40
Chize Lu 5	Kongzui Lu 6	

Xu in Nature

Feishu UB 13	Shanzhong Ren 17	Zusanli St 36
Gaohuang UB 43	Taixi K 3	

Points According to Symptoms

For *palpitations* add Neiquan (P 6).

For *fever* add Quchi (LI 11) and Hegu (LI 4).

The Reasons for Point Selection

Feishu, Fengmen, Taiyuan and Chize all remove obstruction in fei-lung and tonify the fei-lung.

Tiantu and Shanzong relax the chest (bronchodilation).

Zusanli and Gaohuang are points of general tonification.

Hegu and Quchi decrease fever and remove heat.

Fenglong resolves damp.

Taixi tonifies the shen-kidney.

Dingchuan stops the cough and tonifies the fei-lung.

Moxa or cupping should be used on back points as this will alleviate the attacks, control their severity and also decrease the frequency of acute asthmatic attacks.

Auricular Therapy
Dingchuan, lung, adrenal.

Hand Acupuncture
Asthma.

TONSILLITIS

This is due to invasion of wind and heat. The throat is the pathway to the stomach so when there is an infection of the throat there is invasion of wind and heat in the stomach.

Wind and Heat
This is of abrupt onset, there is a fever, thirst, swollen red tonsils and an obvious sore throat. The tongue coating is thin and yellow, the tongue proper red and the pulse is floating and rapid.

Flaring of the Fire of the Stomach
This presents with dysphagia and a yellow-white exudate scattered in spots or flecks on the tonsils. The tongue coating is yellow and greasy, the pulse is rapid.

Treatment
In wind and heat dispel the wind, cool the heat and decrease the swelling and pain. When there is fire of the stomach remove the heat from the stomach, dispel the wind and remove toxins. Use the reducing method in both cases.

Prescription

Wind and Heat
Shaoshang Lu 11   Hegu LI 4   Tianrong SI 17

Flaring of the Fire of the Stomach
Shaoshang Lu 11   Hegu LI 4   Neiting St 44

Points According to Symptoms
For *fever* add Quchi (LI 11).

For *purulent tonsillitis* add Neiting (St 44).

The Reasons for Point Selection
Shaoshang removes heat from the fei-lung and clears the throat.

Tianrong stops pain.

Hegu decreases the swelling and pain.

Neiting removes heat from the stomach.

Quchi disperses heat.

When puncturing Tianrong use a one inch needle towards the root of the tongue, needling sensation must be felt in the throat.

Auricular Therapy
Helix 1-6, Tonsil, Pharynx (use one or two tender spots on Helix).

ACUTE AND CHRONIC RHINITIS AND SINUSITIS

Acute Rhinitis
This is the common cold with associated nasal obstruction and acute inflammation of the nasal cavities. It is caused by the invasion of wind and heat, or wind and cold, frequently after a sudden change of weather.

If there is a deficiency of qi in the fei-lung then the nose, the orifice of the fei-lung, is liable to invasion by pathogens such as wind, heat and cold.

Wind and Cold

This presents with severe nasal obstruction, clear watery discharge and swollen nasal membranes.

Wind and Heat

This presents with a high fever, a purulent nasal discharge, headache and dark yellow urine. The tongue coating is yellow, the tongue proper is red and the pulse is large and rapid.

Treatment

In wind and cold dispel the pathogens and free the nasal passages. Use the reducing method.

In wind and heat clear the heat. Use the reducing method.

Chronic Rhinitis and Sinusitis

This occurs if there is a deficiency of qi in the fei-lung causing an accumulation of pathogenic factors.

Prescription

Wind and Cold

Yingxiang LI 20	Hegu LI 4	Yintang (Extra)
Lieque Lu 7		

Wind and Heat

Yingxiang LI 20	Hegu LI 4	Quchi LI 11
Yintang (Extra)	Dazhui Du 14	

Chronic Rhinitis and Sinusitis

Yingxiang LI 20	Hegu LI 4	Feishu UB 13
Yintang (Extra)	Gaohuang UB 43	

Points According to Symptoms

For *headache* add Taiyang (Extra).

For *frontal sinusitis* add Zanzhu (UB 2).

For *maxillary sinusitis* add Quanliao (SI 18).

The Reasons for Point Selection

Hegu, Yingxiang and Lieque eliminate the pathogens and free nasal cavity.

Yintang strengthens the above function.

Quchi and Dazhui clear heat.

Feishu and Gaohuang free the fei-lung and invigorate the qi of fei-lung.

Auricular Therapy

External nose, internal nose, lung.

HYPERTENSION

Prolonged mental depression, anger and emotional disturbance will lead to depression of qi and hyperactivity of the yang of gan-liver. This in turn will lead to exhaustion of yin fluid.

In senile people, or those with xu of yin of gan-liver and shen-kidney, there will be hyperactivity of yang.

In obese people the function of pi-spleen will be disturbed and there will be an excess of phlegm and damp.

Hyperactivity of Yang

This presents with vertigo, headache, dizziness and irritability. The tongue coating is thin and yellow and the pulse is bowstring and forceless.

Hypoactivity of Yin Leading to Hyperactivity of Yang

This presents with dizziness, tinnitus, headache, blurred vision, a lumbar ache, generalized weakness and insomnia. The tongue proper is red, the pulse is bowstring, fine and rapid.

Excess of Phlegm and Damp

This presents with vertigo, palpitations, a fullness of the chest and epigastrium, nausea and a heavy feeling in the body. The tongue coating is thick and greasy, the pulse is bowstring and gliding.

Treatment

In hyperactivity of yang and hypoactivity of yin pacify the yang of the gan-liver and tonify the yin of shen-kidney. In phlegm and damp strengthen the pi-spleen and resolve damp.

Prescription

Hyperactivity of Yang

Taichong Liv 3   Taixi K 3   Fengchi GB 20
Ganshu UB 18

Hypoactivity of Yin

Taichong Liv 3   Taixi K3   Shenshu UB 23
Sanyinjiao Sp 6

Excess of Phlegm and Damp

Taichong Liv 3   Taixi K 3   Fenglong St 40

Points According to Symptoms

For a *high blood pressure* use Quchi (LI 11) and Zusanli (St 36).

For *palpitations* add Neiguan (P 6).

For *insomnia* add Shenmen (H 7).

For *headache* add Taiyang (Extra).

The Reasons for Point Selection

Taichong and Taixi pacify yang and tonify yin.

Ganshu and Fengchi pacify the fire of the gan-liver.

Shenshu and Sanyinjiao regulate and tonify the shen-kidney and the three yin channels.

Fenglong resolves phlegm in the pi-spleen.

Auricular Therapy

For *lowering the blood pressure* use Groove for lowering the blood pressure and hypertension.

For *dizziness* use Occiput and Forehead.

For *Palpitations* use Heart and Shenmen.

Point Hypertension on the ear can lower the blood pressure smoothly. The rebound increase of blood pressure after treatment is not as rapid as when the Groove for lowering blood pressure is used. When the Groove is used beware of a rapid fall in blood pressure and subsequent hypotension.

CORONARY HEART DISEASE

Coronary heart disease is caused by emotional disturbance, improper intake of food (including over-indulgence) and a lack of exercise.

Shi Type: Retardation of Blood and Stagnation of Qi
This presents with paroxysmal attacks of angina with a fixed painful area, usually in the left shoulder, but in severe cases in the whole back. There may also be excessive sweating, cold extremities, pallor and cyanosis. The tongue proper is purple and the tongue coating is thin and white, with a bowstring or intermittent pulse.

Shi Type: Obstruction by Phlegm and Stagnant Blood
This presents with a stuffy suffocating feeling in the chest and paroxysmal attacks of angina. The tongue proper is purplish, the tongue coating is white and greasy and the pulse is bowstring and gliding.

Xu Type: Xu of Yin of Gan-liver and Shen-kidney
This presents with dizziness, lumbar soreness, thirst and stuffiness in the chest. The tongue coating is thin, the pulse is bowstring and thready.

Xu Type: Xu of Yang of Xin-heart and Shen-kidney
This presents with palpitations, dyspnoea, paroxysmal angina, lumbar soreness, malaise, pallor and peripheral cyanosis. The tongue proper is light or dark purple and the pulse is deep and thready.

Treatment
In the shi types invigorate the circulation of qi and blood, resolve

stasis and remove the obstruction to the channels.

In xu types tonify the deficiency, invigorate the blood circulation of qi and remove the obstruction to the channels.

Prescription

Shi Types
Shanzong Ren 17   Ximen P 4   Neiguan P 6
Jueyinshu UB 14
For stagnation of blood add Geshu (UB 17)
For phlegm add Fenglong (St 40)

Xu Types

Xu of Gan-liver and Shen-kidney
Ganshu UB 18   Shenshu UB 23   Neiguan P 6
Sanyinjiao Sp 6   Shanzong Ren 17

Xu of Yang of Xin-heart and Shen-kidney
Jueyinshu UB 14   Shenshu UB 23   Neiguan P 6
Taixi K 3   Qihai Ren 6

Points According to Symptoms
For *acute angina* use Ximen (P 4).

The Reasons for Point Selection
Shanzong invigorates the circulation of qi and blood.

Jueyinshu, Neiguan and Ximen resolve stasis and remove obstruction.

Ganshu, Shenshu and Sanyinjiao tonify the gan-liver and shen-kidney.

Fenglong resolves phlegm.

Geshu invigorates blood circulation.

ACUTE CONJUNCTIVITIS

This is caused by wind and heat invading the eye and resulting in a red, painful purulent eye.

Treatment
Clear wind and heat.

Prescription

Hegu LI 4	Taiyang (Extra)	Jingming UB 1
Foot-linqi GB 41		

The Reasons for Point Selection
Jingming and Taiyang remove heat.

Hegu removes heat and inflammation.

Foot-linqi is therapeutically successful.

URTICARIA

This is caused by wind and heat, or wind and cold, invading the skin and muscles. This causes impairment of the circulation of qi and blood, and the extravasation of blood. The onset of the rash is abrupt.

Wind and Cold
The rash is pale pink and is relieved by warmth.

Wind and Heat
The rash is red, hot and itchy.

Treatment
In wind and cold, dispel the wind and clear cold.

In wind and heat, dispel the wind and clear heat.

Prescription

Wind and Cold

Quchi LI 11	Hegu LI 4	Lieque Lu 7
Sanyinjiao Sp 6		

Wind and Heat

Quchi LI 11	Hegu LI 4	Lieque Lu 7
Sanyinjiao Sp 6	Xuehai Sp 10	Geshu UB 17

Points According to Symptoms

Add Zusanli (St 36) and Shangjuxu (St 37) if there is *gastric involvement*.

The Reasons for Point Selection

Hegu and Quchi remove wind.

Xuehai and Geshu remove heat and help to relieve the itching.

Sanyinjiao tonifies the yin.

Lieque dispels wind and tonifies the fei-lung.

D. MISCELLANEOUS DISEASES

ACUTE SIMPLE APPENDICITIS

Immoderate and excessive eating and drinking causes a functional disturbance of the intestine which allows the invasion of damp and heat, and this causes retardation of qi and stagnation of blood. The tongue coating is yellow or greasy and the pulse normal or rapid.

Treatment
Cool the heat and remove the obstruction by promoting the circulation of qi and blood.

Prescription
Lanwei (Extra)　　　　Shangjuxu St 37　　　　Zusanli St 36
Tianshu St 25

Points According to Symptoms
For *fever* add Quchi (LI 11) and Hegu (LI 4).

For *nausea* add Neiguan (P 6).

The Reasons for Point Selection
Lanwei is effective. Seventy per cent to eighty per cent of patients who have appendicitis have tenderness at Lanwei, or another point nearby. Lanwei is punctured bilaterally.

Tianshu regulates the function of the intestine and cools the heat.

Zusanli, Quchi and Hegu remove heat.

Neiguan regulates the function of the stomach.

Treat twice to four times a day in the acute stage leaving the needles in for about an hour, and manipulate them every fifteen minutes. Continue treatment for a week or so after the initial diagnosis, gradually tailing off treatment according to symptoms. If there is no improvement in the first twenty-four hours then a laparotomy is mandatory.

TOOTHACHE

Toothache may be due to either exogenous pathogens or endogenous factors. The endogenous factors are xu of shen-kidney or a blazing up of the fire of the stomach. The endogenous weakness may be affected by exogenous factors. Invasion of wind in the stomach channel can turn into fire. The intake of sour or sweet foods, when there is xu of shen-kidney, may also aggravate toothache.

Shi Type (abscess-fire)
This presents with continuous painful toothache, a foul smell in the mouth, fever and swelling in the local area. The tongue coating is thin and yellow, the pulse is bowstring and gliding.

Xu Type (cavity-kidney)
This presents with vague intermittent pain, lassitude and a lumbar ache. The tooth is loose, the tongue coating is thin and white and the pulse is thready and forceless.

Treatment
In shi type, clear the heat and reduce the fire.

In xu type, reinforce and tonify the qi of shen-kidney.

Prescription

Shi Type
Xiaguan St 7	Hegu LI 4	Jiache St 6
Neiting St 44		

Xu Type
Shenshu UB 23	Taixi K 3	Hegu LI 4
Neiting St 44		

Points According to Symptoms
For a *lower jaw ache* use Neiting (St 44), for an upper jaw ache use Hegu (LI 4).

For *headache* add Fengchi (GB 20).

For *fever* add Waiguan (SJ 5).

The Reasons for Point Selection

Neiting, Xiaguan and Jiache clear fire and remove the obstruction in the channels.

Taixi and Shenshu reinforce the shen-kidney.

Fengchi and Waiguan eliminate wind and heat.

Hegu is the source point of the affected channel.

Auricular Therapy

Lower/upper toothache, Shenmen, Tragic apex.

Hand Acupuncture

Yatong (Extra).

DYSMENORRHOEA

Cold

If the patient gets cold, or eats too much cold food, the cold stops normal circulation of qi and dysmenorrhoea results. This presents with pain and a cold feeling in the lower abdomen, with the pain improving when it is warmed. There are dark red clots in the menstrual discharge, the tongue coating is thin and white and the pulse is deep and slow, or bowstring.

Retardation of Qi of the Gan-liver

Persistent depression or irritability retards the qi of the gan-liver, and also causes dysmenorrhoea. This presents with severe abdominal pain, distension in both flanks and distension of the breasts and in the costal region. The menstrual fluid is purple and there are large clots in it. The tongue has a dark red coating with purple spots and the pulse is deep and bowstring.

Treatment

In cold, dispel cold and warm, therefore freeing the Ren channel. In retardation of qi, regulate qi and eliminate the stagnant blood.

Prescription

Guanyuan Ren 4   Taichong Liv 3   Sanyinjiao Sp 6
Shiquizhui (Extra)

The Reasons for Point Selection
Sanyinjiao and Guanyuan warm the channels and relieve pain.

Shiqizhui frees the channels.

Taichong regulates the function of the gan-liver.

Treat once a day to relieve symptoms. If treatment is to be used to prevent pain then treat daily for the five to seven days prior to a period.

MORNING SICKNESS

Only treat morning sickness if it is severe. During pregnancy the qi and blood are directed to the Ren and Chong channels. This nourishes the baby but it can lead to a lack of qi and blood in the rest of the body. The excess of qi in the Ren and Chong channels can invade the Stomach channel and cause vomiting.

Treatment
Regulate the stomach and pi-spleen and stop the vomiting.

Prescription
Neiguan P 6   Gongsun Sp 4   Zusanli St 36

The Reasons for Point Selection
Neiguan controls the middle jiao. (This contains the stomach and pi-spleen.)

Zusanli regulates the stomach.

Gongsun connects with the chong channel to regulate the pi-spleen and stomach.

MENOPAUSAL SYMPTOMS

Prescription
Sanyinjiao Sp 6   Gongsun Sp 4   Taichong Liv 3
Neiguan P 6

The Reasons for Point Selection

Sanyinjiao and Gongsun stop vomiting and help dizziness.

Taichong and Neiguan stop palpitations and hot flushes.

Auricular Therapy

Endocrine, Uterus, Shenmen.

Give two courses, the first daily and the second on alternate days.

MODERN ACUPUNCTURE METHODS

EAR ACUPUNCTURE

The ear is a homunculus with all of the structures and organs of the body represented on it. The origin of ear acupuncture is unclear, and although it is referred to in ancient Chinese texts it only seems to have been used clinically during the last fifty years.

In broad principle the apex of the pinna represents the hands and feet, the helix and anti-helix the limbs and trunk, the ear lobe the facial structures, and the concha of the ear represents the internal organs. The main auricular points are shown on the ear chart.

Ear acupuncture can be used for any condition that will respond to acupuncture, although in China its main use is for acutely painful conditions and acupuncture anaesthesia.

I.   POINT SELECTION

The Theory of Point Selection

Auricular points can be selected directly for the areas they represent; stomach point for gastralgia, ankle point for ankle pain, and so on. They can also be selected on the basis of traditional Chinese medicine, for instance when there is a disturbance of the gan-liver select the liver point, or for diseases of the skin select the lung point as the fei-lung controls the skin and hair.

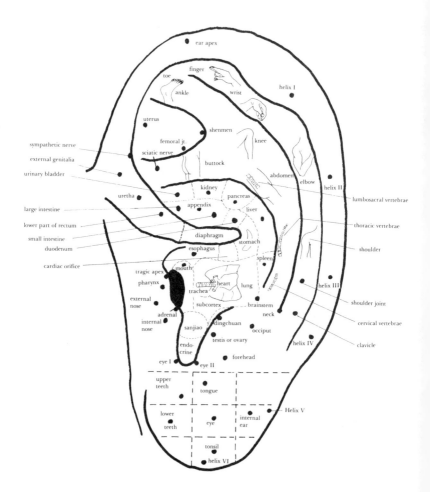

The Anterior of the Ear.

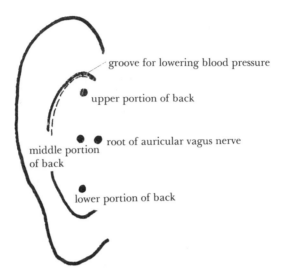

The Posterior of the Ear.

The Chinese were also selecting points on the basis of modern physiology, for instance in gynaecological problems endocrine and subcortex points are frequently used. Some of the points are based on clinical experience, Shenmen is a useful sedative point Dingchuan is useful for asthma, and Appendix for appendicitis.

Methods of Point Selection

In ear acupuncture it is essential to localize the ear points accurately. If a structure or organ in the body is painful or diseased then the ear point representing that organ will be painful. This can be demonstrated clinically by probing the ear; initially the acupuncturist must decide on the approximate area to probe and then carefully search the area with a blunt probe or a spring-loaded probe. The point that is the most painful is the one that requires treatment.

Ear points can also be localized electrically. A tender ear point has an increased electrical conductance and, by using one of the many electrical ear point locators that are available, the area of

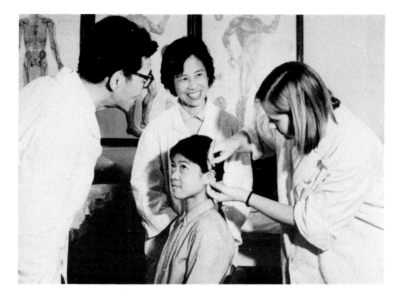

Probing the Ear to Locate an Acupuncture Point.

increased conductance can be demonstrated. These machines are very prone to artefact so the operator must use them with extreme care and not press on the ear too forcefully or areas of increased conduction will appear everywhere.

Point Selection for Pain
In acute pain ear acupuncture can have a very swift and effective action. The point should be selected by the methods described. When the needle is inserted into the tender point the patient will feel a great deal of pain. Rotate the needle and get the patient to exercise the painful area at the same time. The pain in the affected area should then disappear.

Chronic pain may also respond quite dramatically to ear acupuncture, but to be effective it may often require a course of treatment rather than one treatment.

II. NEEDLING TECHNIQUE

Sterility
It is important to keep ear needles sterile and to clean the ear carefully before inserting a needle.

Needle Insertion
Half inch or one inch needles should be used in the ear. The half inch needles can be inserted perpendicularly to the skin and the one inch needles are often used obliquely. Do not insert the needle through the ear. Press studs can also be used in the ear. They are useful for chronic conditions as the patient can press the stud and stimulate the point whenever symptoms occur.

Needle Stimulation
Ear points can be stimulated manually by rotating the needle; this creates a burning painful sensation in the ear. Electrical stimulation of the ear points is used to induce anaesthesia and it can also be used therapeutically, especially in chronic conditions. The main use of the electrical stimulator in China is for ear acupuncture anaesthesia. The stimulation frequencies used were usually low for any form of ear acupuncture, between 5 and 300Hz, but there seemed to be no consistent agreement about the exact frequency. The intensity used is the maximum tolerable.

III. AURICULAR THERAPY

Ear point prescriptions have been included in the sections, where relevant, on each particular disease.

Ear acupuncture should be treated like body acupuncture for chronic conditions; the patient should be given a course of about eight treatments, although acute conditions may respond in one treatment.

SCALP ACUPUNCTURE

Scalp acupuncture is a modern acupuncture method. The Chinese attribute its development to Chiao Sun-Fa, a 35-year-old physician in North China, and it has been used in China since 1971. The principle of scalp acupuncture is very straightforward; the aim is to stimulate the diseased area of the brain in order to facilitate a return of function in that area.

This method is based on elementary functional neuro-anatomy, and has nothing to do with traditional Chinese medicine. If part of the brain is damaged, for instance by a stroke, then the scalp is stimulated over the damaged area of the brain. All the scalp points are representations of the underlying functional areas of the brain. It therefore follows that the most common use of scalp acupuncture will be in diseases in which there is brain damage, such as strokes or severe head injuries, although this method can be used for a variety of other conditions. Scalp acupuncture is particularly useful for reducing chronic muscle spasm.

I. LOCALIZATION OF SCALP POINTS

When using scalp therapy it is vital to localize the scalp area accurately. There are very few good reference texts for such scalp points so accurate scalp maps have been included in this text.

TABLE V.

Area	Localization	Use
Motor area	0.5cms posterior to the midpoint of the anterior-posterior line defines the upper limit of the motor area. The lower limit intersects the eyebrow-occiput line at the anterior border of the natural hairline on the temple. The upper 1/5 represents the lower limbs and trunk, the middle 2/5 represents the upper limbs and the lower 2/5 the face.	Contralateral motor disturbance of the appropriate area.

Area	Localization	Use
Sensory area	This is a line parallel to the motor area and 1.5cms behind it. The sensory input to the lower limbs and trunk is represented on the upper 1/5, the middle 2/5 represents the upper limbs, and the lower 2/5 represents the face.	Contralateral sensory disturbances of the appropriate area, pain and vertigo.
Foot motor-sensory area	Parallel to and 1cm lateral to the anterior-posterior line. The line is 3cms long and starts 1cm posterior to the line representing the sensory area.	Motor and sensory disturbances of the lower limbs and genito-urinary system.
Chorea-tremor area	Parallel to and 1.5cms in front of the motor area.	Parkinson's disease and tremor and chorea from any cause.
Vasomotor area	Parallel to and 1.5cms in front of the chorea-tremor area.	Cerebral oedema and hypertension.
Vertigo-auditory area	A 4cm horizontal line with its centre located 1.5cms above the apex of the pinna.	Tinnitus, vertigo and deafness.
1st Speech or usage area	Taking the parietal tubercule as a reference point insert three needles separately at 40° to each other. Each line is 3cms long.	Parietal lobe lesions.
2nd Speech area	This line is 3cms long and starts on a point 2cms posterior-inferior to the parietal tubercule and parallel to the anterior-posterior line.	Nominal aphasia.
3rd Speech area	A 4cms line originating at the midpoint of the vertigo-auditory area and running posteriorly.	Sensory aphasia.

Area	Localization	Use
Optic area	This area originates 1cm lateral to the midpoint of the occipital protruberance and runs for 4cms parallel to the anterior-posterior line in an anterior direction.	Cortical blindness.
Balance area	This area originates 3cms lateral to the midpoint of the occipital protruberance and runs for 4cms parallel to the anterior-posterior line in a posterior direction.	Cerebellar disease.
Gastric area	A line directly above the pupil starting from the hairline and running for 2cms in a posterior direction parallel to the anterior-posterior line.	Epigastric discomfort.
Thoracic area	Midway between the anterior-posterior midline and the gastric area. It is a 4cms line with its midpoint on the hairline, running parallel to the gastric area.	Respiratory and cardio-vascular diseases.
Repro-duction area	A 2cms line parallel to the gastric area originating at the hair line and running posteriorly. The thoracic area and reproduction area originate at points equidistant from the gastric area.	Uterine haemorrhage.

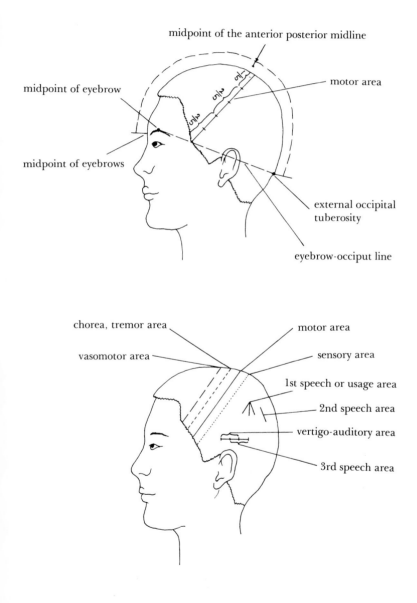

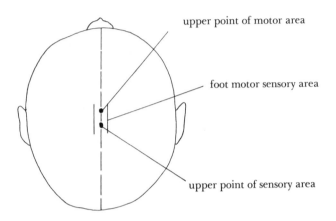

upper point of motor area

foot motor sensory area

upper point of sensory area

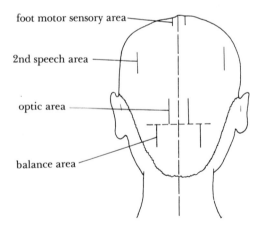

foot motor sensory area

2nd speech area

optic area

balance area

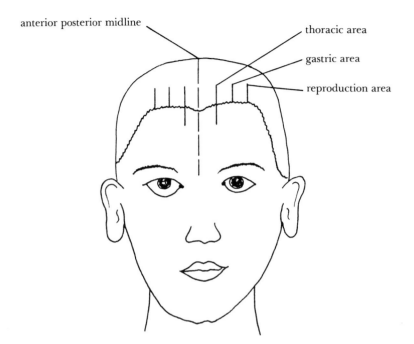

anterior posterior midline

thoracic area

gastric area

reproduction area

II. NEEDLING TECHNIQUE

Skin Sterility
It is important to sterilize the skin before inserting the needle. The Chinese use a solution of 2.5% iodine and 75% alcohol to do this. Hair is not usually a problem and it can be parted to expose the scalp, but if long-term scalp therapy is required then it may be easier to shave the scalp area.

Needle Insertion
The Chinese usually insert a 2-inch or 3-inch needle into the scalp area, running it down the subcutaneous layer. This requires a great deal of dexterity with an acupuncture needle and it is easier to use several short consecutively connecting needles over the scalp area.

Needle Stimulation
The needle should be rotated without any lifting and thrusting

movement. In general the more a scalp area is stimulated the better is the result, the Chinese recommending that the needle be rotated manually at a frequency greater than 200 times per minute for about five minutes. This should be repeated two or three times during a twenty to thirty minutes period of treatment. Many Chinese use electrical stimulation over the scalp areas, the stimulator being used at high frequency (about 3000Hz), and maximum tolerable intensity, for about twenty minutes. When the scalp is stimulated the patient often feels a burning sensation in the scalp and a dull, numb or distended feeling in the relevant area.

Selection of Scalp Areas

In order to know which scalp areas should be stimulated a clear neurological diagnosis must be made. The contralateral area is usually stimulated, but better results seem to be obtained if the area is stimulated bilaterally.

III. THE INDICATIONS FOR THE USE OF SCALP ACUPUNCTURE

Routine medical management should always be carried out first, and if scalp acupuncture is indicated then it should be used to aid recovery and deal with the chronic sequelae.

Cerebro-vascular Accidents

Scalp acupuncture is particularly useful in all types of strokes, whether the origin is cerebral thrombus or a cerebral haemorrhage. Do not start scalp needling for at least a week after the stroke; scalp acupuncture increases the blood flow to the damaged area of the brain and local cerebral bleeding may be increased if it is used too early. Scalp acupuncture can be started up to two years after the onset of a stroke, with beneficial results.

Prescription
Use the relevant scalp area; if there is motor pathology in a specific area then use the relevant motor area. This rule applies to all pathology, therefore a clear neurological diagnosis of which area(s) is affected is essential.

The contralateral area on the scalp must be used but, in general, better results are obtained if the affected area is stimulated bilaterally.

Treatment
Sometimes strokes respond very quickly, but not always. It may be necessary to give several courses of scalp acupuncture. As with all types of acupuncture keep treating the patient as long as there is improvement, and then give a few more treatments to consolidate. Each course involves about eight treatments and there should be a gap of at least a week between courses. The treatments should be given daily or every other day.

Severe Head Injuries
Follow the same rules of treatment and prescription as for cerebro-vascular accidents. Scalp acupuncture is particularly useful for reducing chronic muscle spasm. Treat after routine medical treatment when the patient's condition is stable.

Intracranial Inflammation
After routine medical treatment is completed, and the patient's condition is stable, treat the areas that are damaged. Follow the same rules for treatment and prescription as for cerebro-vascular accidents.

Extra-Pyramidal Disease
Chorea and paralysis agitans are the main extra-pyramidal diseases. The most important scalp area is the chorea-tremor area. Parkinson's syndrome responds better than Parkinson's disease. Follow the same rules for treatment and prescription as for cerebro-vascular accidents.

Suggestions for Other Diseases

Disease	*Area*
Meniere's syndrome	Bilateral vertigo-auditory area
Respiratory diseases	Bilateral thoracic area
Gastric diseases	Bilateral gastric area
Urticaria	Bilateral upper 1/5 of the sensory area

Cardiovascular disease   Bilateral thoracic area

Cerebral oedema   Bilateral vasomotor area

IV. CONCLUSION

Scalp acupuncture is useful for a wide variety of diseases, especially those of cortical origin. It is most useful for strokes and severe head injuries, but it should always be considered for other conditions where other methods of acupuncture are failing to give adequate results. It is particularly useful in reducing chronic muscle spasticity.

HAND ACUPUNCTURE

This is used primarily for acute conditions such as back strain or acute torticollis. The points are selected on a purely symptomatic basis. It is essential to obtain deqi over these points and, especially for acute conditions, to stimulate the hand points strongly. This can be very painful for the patient, who may faint.

Where hand acupuncture is useful the relevant point(s) is mentioned in the section on diseases. The hand points should be stimulated strongly whilst the patient exercises the painful area. It may be necessary to stimulate the hand points for some minutes, although the relief of pain and muscle spasm is often immediate.

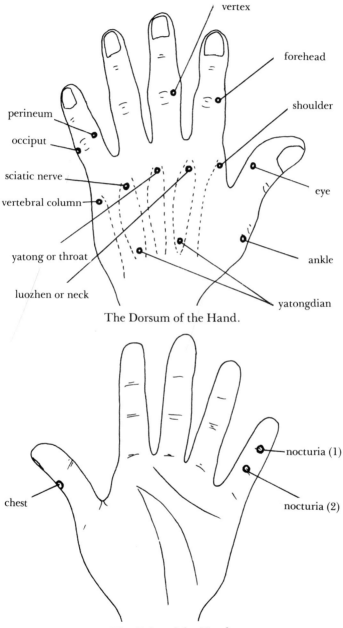

The Dorsum of the Hand.

The Palm of the Hand.

ACUPUNCTURE ANAESTHESIA AND THE PHYSIOLOGICAL BASIS OF ACUPUNCTURE

ACUPUNCTURE ANAESTHESIA

Acupuncture anaesthesia is a recent and purely Chinese invention. The Thoughts of Chairman Mao state that 'Chinese medicine and pharmacology are a great treasure house and efforts should be made to explore them and raise them to a higher level.' This was a very important impetus to the development of this application of acupuncture.

The Chinese look upon acupuncture anaesthesia as a useful working method for local or regional anaesthesia. They do not consider their methods of acupuncture anaesthesia to be perfect, but they look upon it as a subject that is being evaluated and developed all the time. The majority of operative procedures in Chinese hospitals are done with local or regional anaesthetics, and acupuncture anaesthesia is probably the commonest form of regional anaesthetic in use. Most hospitals that we visited seemed to be using acupuncture anaesthesia for between 40% and 60% of their surgical procedures.

The use of acupuncture anaesthesia is not confined to minor operations but includes major abdominal and cardio-thoracic surgery. During our visit to China we saw more than forty operations with acupuncture as the anaesthetic. There is no doubt that it was effective in a wide variety of operations. The Chinese often give figures of about 90% success rate, but our impression was that it was an acceptable form of anaesthesia for nearly all the operations we saw.

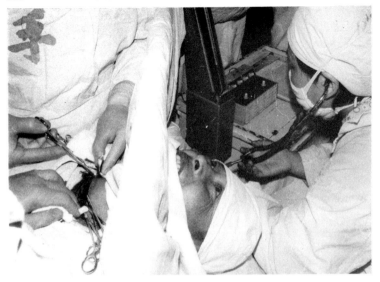

Acupuncture Anaesthesia: A Thyroid Operation.

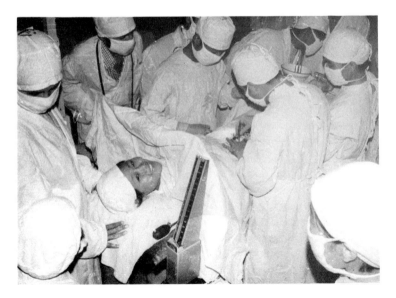

Acupuncture Anaesthesia: An Appendicectomy.

The clinical advantages of acupuncture anaesthesia are obvious. It is a safe and considerably less dangerous procedure than general anaesthesia, it is safer for the old and disabled, post-operative recovery is far swifter, it is a very cheap and simple form of anaesthesia, and the physiological functions of the body, such as the pulse rate and blood pressure, remain consistently stable during anaesthesia. The main disadvantage is that very occasionally the anaesthetic does not work and an alternative form of anaesthesia may be required fairly swiftly.

The possibility that a small number of patients might experience some pain is probably unacceptable in the context of a Western medical system. Furthermore, there is no muscle relaxation in acupuncture anaesthesia so it can be quite hard work to retract the abdominal muscles. Also, the Chinese have not found a solution to the discomfort that is occasionally caused by traction on the visceral contents.

Before acupuncture anaesthesia the Chinese explain to the patients what is going to happen. Most people, including the Chinese, are very frightened before going into an operating theatre, especially if they are going to be awake. It is therefore important to have the confidence of the patient before embarking on any type of surgery involving local anaesthesia. A pre-medication of barbiturates is usually given and the patient is wheeled to theatre. Body and ear points are selected on the same basis as for therapy and these are then stimulated electrically. In general low frequencies are used on the ear points and on distal body points (5-300Hz), and high frequencies are used on local points (3000-10,000Hz). When using the body points deqi is obtained first. When using ear points the Chinese insert the needle obliquely to be sure of hitting the point, and tape the needle in. Ear points will not be painful because there is not usually any local pain pre-operatively.

A period of induction is required whether ear or body points are used, and this is usually about twenty minutes. After inserting the needles the electrical stimulator is connected, set at the required frequency and maximum tolerable intensity, and left on throughout the operation. After the induction period anaesthesia should be adequate for the operation. For particularly painful operative procedures, such as separating the periosteum from the bone, small amounts of local anaesthetic are sometimes used. Very occasionally intravenous narcotics may be given if the operation is prolonged or the procedure is painful.

Point selection for acupuncture anaesthesia follows exactly the same rules as acupuncture therapy. When seleching body points for a thyroidectomy use Hegu (LI 4) and Neiguan (P 6) as distathe same rules as acupuncture therapy. When selecting body points for a thyroidectomy use Hegu (LI 4) and Neiguan (P 6) as distal points, and Neck-Futu (LI 18) as a local point. The ear points for this operation would be Throat, Neck, Shenmen and Subcortex; Throat and Neck are local points and Shenmen and Subcortex are sedative points. It is obvious, therefore, that the principles of point selection follow the principles of point selection for therapy, i.e. when using body acupuncture select local and distal points and when using ear acupuncture select local representative points and add in sedative points.

Acupuncture anaesthesia is a fascinating application of acupuncture; perhaps, in the West, it could be used for post-operative analgesia rather than anaesthesia.

SOME IDEAS ON THE PHYSIOLOGICAL BASIS OF ACUPUNCTURE

At present there is no unified theory that explains the complex mechanism of acupuncture, but there are many well substantiated physiological changes that do occur when this technique is applied. The Chinese are investing a large amount of research resources in the investigation of the physiology of acupuncture; they are not limited to the traditional approach but they do see that this is empirically useful and gives better results than simply needling tender areas. Contradictions can co-exist easily in the Chinese mind and so there is no real conflict between the traditional and the more scientific approach to acupuncture, and furthermore they see this combined approach as mutually beneficial.

Acupuncture points are well known to us in the West, studies by Melzack show that acupuncture points correlate very closely with trigger points[1] and that the use of these trigger points, particularly for injection therapy, is a well recognized technique within

Western medicine. These tender areas (acupuncture points) are frequently to be found on or near neuromuscular junctions. Further work by Becker also strongly suggests that acupuncture points have special electrical properties, and that the skin over acupuncture points is able to pass electrical current more easily than the surrounding areas of normal skin.[2] As yet, however, there is no good anatomical or physiological basis for the theory of the channels; although a considerable amount of physiological investigation has been directed at attempting to prove the existence of channels.[3]

The fact that acupuncture works as an analgesic is quite clear; surgical analgesia in animals and in man follows the needling of specific acupuncture points, and sham needling of non-specific points does not produce analgesia.[4] Furthermore, using the human model of dental pain, acupuncture can also be shown to be a specific and relatively powerful analgesic. However, there has been a distinct lack of good clinical trials on the effect of acupuncture as a therapy for chronic pain problems; the author has reviewed the studies that are available and suggested models that can be used for the clinical evaluation of acupuncture.[6] Such clinical trials are essential if acupuncture is to progress as a therapeutic technique within the context of Western medicine.

When an acupuncture point is stimulated various neurological and neurohumoral changes occur in the body. In decerebrate cats, stimulation of the skin inhibits the passage of painful stimuli.[7] Work on small animals also shows that stimulating a specific acupuncture point changes the nerve transmission in the painful area, the spinal cord and the thalamus.[8] Furthermore, some of the detailed neurophysiological studies completed at the Shanghai Institute of Physiology suggests that there is a supra-spinal centre that inhibits viscerosomatic reflexes and that this is stimulated via acupuncture points; there is considerable evidence which would support the mediation of painful stimuli at a thalamic level as being one of the important mechanisms through which acupuncture can have an effect.[9]

The gate theory of pain[10] also goes some way to explain the mechanism of acupuncture in pain. All pain input enters the spinal cord via the substantia gelatinosa, pain impulses travelling along the small nerve fibres. The large myelenated nerve fibres have an inhibitory effect on pain, by closing the gate to pain at cordal level, within the substantia gelatinosa. If pain is not transmitted to the brain, no pain is perceived. Melzack has suggested that acupuncture stimulates large myelenated nerve fibres, thereby closing the gate to pain.[11] However, there are a large number of problems with the gate theory of pain, particularly it is used to explain the mechanism of acupuncture. It is probable that acupuncture does work partially through the gate control theory, although this cannot be seen as a complete explanation of its mechanism.

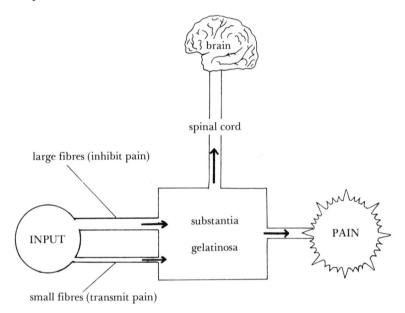

The Gate Theory of Pain.

Endorphins, or naturally occurring morphine-like substances, have recently been found in a wide variety of body tissues. In people suffering from chronic pain the endorphin level in the fluid around the brain, the cerebrospinal fluid, is low. Acupuncture increases the endorphin level in various parts of the central nervous system and β-endorphin can be shown to attenuate chronic pain.[12] This analgesic effect can sometimes be blocked by naloxone, a morphine antagonist,[13] although other studies suggest that the analgesic effect of acupuncture cannot be reversed by naloxone. Therefore, although the endorphin theory is another very useful idea through which acupuncture can be shown to have an effect, it does not seem to explain the complete physiological mechanism of this therapeutic technique.

These two ideas, the gate control theory of pain and endorphins, are not mutually exclusive. They go some way towards explaining the possible mechanism of acupuncture in pain, but the clinical application of acupuncture is much wider than its use in pain, so these ideas leave a great deal unexplained..

During our course we had a considerable number of lectures on the physiological basis of acupuncture, and some interesting ideas were discussed. As well as having an analgesic effect acupuncture seems to have a sedative effect. Puncturing Zusanli (St 36) bilaterally caues the alpha rhythm in the brain to predominate, and its amplitude to increase. Acupuncture also has a regulatory and anti-shock effect, which has been clearly demonstrated by creating massive blood loss in dogs; the dogs receiving acupuncture show a significantly increased survival rate![14] Acupuncture also affects the immune system; needling increases the white cell count, raises the titres of all groups of immunoglobulins, increases the activity of the reticulo-endothelial system and raises the level of serum complement. The claims that acupuncture can affect the immune system have been made primarily by the Chinese, but the author has also conducted some preliminary research which would seem to confirm this hypothesis. Furthermore, acupuncture has been shown, quite clearly, to cause changes in many of the chemical messengers (neurotransmitters) within many different areas of the brain.[15]

This short summary of the available evidence strongly suggests that acupuncture is having a fundamental physiological effect on the human body. The reason for including this section is that the scientific investigation of acupuncture is an integral part of the modern Chinese approach to acupuncture; this brief review just summarizes some of the current ideas in this field and more detailed information, dealing with these and other concepts, is available in many Western scientific journals (particularly the journal *Pain*). The effect of acupuncture on the body is attracting a great deal of scientific interest, both in China and the West. The field is changing fast and progressively more of the empirical findings of the ancient Chinese are being scientifically validated.

REFERENCES

[1] Melzack et al, 1977, *Pain*, 3 (1977), page 3.

[2] Becker et al, *Transactions on Biomedical Engineering*, (1975) page 533.

[3] *National Symposia of Acupuncture Moxibustion and Acupuncture Anaesthesia*, Peking, 1979.

[4] Teral (Doctoral thesis), Faculty of Medicine, Montpellier, (1975).

[5] Chapman et al, *Pain*, 9 (1980), page 183.

[6] Lewith et al, *Pain*, 16 (1983), page 111.

[7] Hill et al, *Experimental Brain Research*, 9 (1969), page 284.

[8] Niboyet et al, *L'Anaesthesic par l'Acupuncture*, Moulins-les-Metz, France, (1973).

[9] Eh Shen et al, *Chinese Medical Journal*, 1 (1975), page 431.

[10] Melzack et al, *Science*, 150 (1965), page 197.

[11] Melzack et al, *Pain*, 1 (1975), page 357.

[12] Akil et al, *Science*, 201 (1978), page 463.

[13] Pomeranz, *Advances in Biomedical Psychopharmacology*, 18, page 351.

[14] Anon, 1974, *Journal of Chinese Medicine*, 2 (1974), page 261.

[15] Han Jisheng, *National Symposia of Acupuncture, Moxibustion and Acupuncture Anaesthesia*. Peking, 1979, page 27.

INDEX